Preparing
for the DRCOG

D1152030

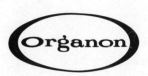
Organon

Presented with the compliments of
Organon Laboratories

Preparing for the DRCOG
MCQs and Case Studies

Janice Rymer, MD, MRCOG, FRNZCOG
Senior Lecturer and Honorary Consultant
Guy's and St Thomas' Hospital, London

and

Jennie Higham, MD, MRCOG, MFFP
Senior Registrar, Luton and Dunstable
and St Mary's Hospital, London

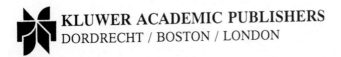 KLUWER ACADEMIC PUBLISHERS
DORDRECHT / BOSTON / LONDON

Every attempt has been made to ensure the accuracy of the information in this book. However, neither Organon Laboratories Ltd nor Kluwer Academic Publishers can accept responsibility for the use of this information.

The help of Jeannie Hughes in the preparation of this book is gratefully acknowledged.

Distributors

for the United States and Canada: Kluwer Academic Publishers, PO Box 358, Accord Station, Hingham, MA 02018-0358, USA
for all other countries: Kluwer Academic Publishers Group, Distribution Center, PO Box 322, 3300 AH Dordrecht, The Netherlands

A catalogue record for this book is available from the British Library.

ISBN 0-7923-8875-5

Contents

Foreword

The Royal College of Obstetricians and Gynaecologists (RCOG) awards a diploma to those registered medical practitioners who have had an appropriate postgraduate training in the subject and who are able to satisfy its examiners. This Diploma is intended to recognize the general practitioner's non-specialist training in obstetrics and gynaecology.

Following a working party report which identified defects in the reliability and validity of the old-style examination, the RCOG has recently amended the methods of assessment. The DRCOG examination now consists of an MCQ paper which covers all areas of obstetrics and gynaecology, along with its associated subjects. Additionally, each candidate participates in an Objective Structured Clinical Examination (OSCE). OSCEs are organized as a series of stations through which each candidate rotates. Individual tasks are set, designed to challenge certain areas of knowledge and competence. The skills assessed include tests of factual information, problem solving, diagnosis, investigation and treatment and communication skills. Performance is judged against pre-set criteria and has the advantage of offering the same examination experience to each candidate. Only a single or small number of trained examiners is involved in each station or task, again adding to the consistency of the OSCE.

This book aims to give the prospective candidate appropriate training in both MCQs and case studies covering a wide range of topics. The case studies have been included to familiarize candidates with the factual and problem-solving approaches now used in the OSCE.

This format allows the candidate to further supplement his or her revision by providing explanations for each answer. Rather than pure reading of facts this should be a welcome alternative and aid the retention of knowledge.

Assessing the work of junior staff is a vital part of ensuring the competence of tomorrow's senior doctors and we hope this revision book demonstrates how relatively painless and enjoyable learning can be!

Janice Rymer   *Jenny Higham*

MCQs: Paper I

1. **Natural menopause**

A. may occur under the age of 35
B. is associated with an increase in HDL cholesterol
C. accelerates bone loss
D. causes an increase in KPI
E. occurs at an average age of 54 in the UK

2. **Secondary amenorrhoea may be due to**

A. thyrotoxicosis
B. virilizing ovarian tumour
C. imperforate hymen
D. Asherman's syndrome
E. endometriosis

3. **Regarding human fertility**

A. fertilization usually occurs 5–7 days before implantation and before the extrusion of the second polar body
B. subfertility is common following mumps in women
C. an adverse male factor is detectable in about 30% of couples with low fertility
D. hyperstimulation syndrome may occur as a complication of GIFT
E. micromanipulation is a treatment for oligospermia

4. **Sterilization**

A. in men has a failure rate of about 1 in 300 cases
B. in men is associated with an increase in coronary heart disease
C. in women prevents ectopic pregnancies
D. in women decreases menstrual loss
E. in women can be successfully reversed if clips were used for the original operation in >80% of cases

5. Regarding thromboembolic disease

A. there is a greater risk in a multiple than in a singleton pregnancy
B. heparin should not be given in the first trimester
C. warfarin increases the likelihood of fetal haemorrhage
D. in pregnancy heparin therapy can cause maternal osteoporosis
E. the risk is increased in women who are blood group O

6. Monozygotic twins

A. are less common than dizygotic twins
B. are commonly familial
C. may be reliably distinguished from dizygotic twins by naked-eye examination studying the fetal membranes and placentae
D. have a higher incidence of placenta praevia than singleton pregnancies
E. are associated with acute polyhydramnios

7. Spina bifida

A. is associated with raised maternal serum α-fetoprotein (AFP) level
B. can be diagnosed by ultrasound scan during the third trimester
C. is inherited as an autosomal recessive
D. is associated with dilated cerebral ventricles
E. screening is part of the triple test

8. In development of the female genital tract

A. the fallopian tubes are derived from the Müllerian ducts
B. the external genitalia can be recognized as male or female by the 18th week of fetal life
C. failure of fusion of the Müllerian ducts results in uterus didelphis
D. the upper third of the vagina is formed from the cloaca
E. Wolffian ducts degenerate in the absence of a Y chromosome

9. In human genetics

A. an XO genotype is associated with male somatotype
B. the total number of chromosomes in both males and females is 48
C. chromatin-positive cells (Barr body present) are characteristic of normal women
D. genetic chorionic villous sampling is associated with a fetal loss of 1%
E. the Y chromosome determines the development of the ovary

10. In the normal cervix

A. the canal is lined by transitional epithelium
B. the mucus is scanty at the time of ovulation
C. the level of the squamo-columnar junction varies at different phases of reproductive life
D. keratinized stratified epithelium is found over the vaginal aspects of the cervix
E. the squamo-columnar junction is usually visible on speculum examination after menopause

11. In the fetal skull

A. the biparietal diameter is approximately 9.5 cm at term
B. the lambdoidal suture runs between the frontal and parietal bones
C. the bregma is the area lying between the parietal and occipital bones
D. the sub-occipito bregmatic diameter is the engaging diameter when the head is fully flexed in a vertex presentation
E. the occiput is the denominator in a vertex presentation

12. In the fetal circulatory system

A. blood flows from fetus to placenta in the umbilical arteries
B. the ductus arteriosus closes during labour
C. placental circulation starts at about 5 weeks gestational age
D. the heart becomes a four-chamber organ at about 7 weeks gestational age
E. reverse and diastolic flow in the umbilical artery is associated with fetal hypoxia

13. The following hormones are secreted within the posterior lobe of the human pituitary gland

A. oxytocin
B. thyroid stimulating hormone
C. luteinizing hormone
D. adrenocorticotrophin
E. prolactin

14. Regarding ovum and spermatozoa

A. the spermatozoa are responsible for at least 10% of the volume of the ejaculate
B. the fertilized ovum has embedded by the 16-cell stage of development
C. the ovum can be fertilized up to 4 days after ovulation
D. human spermatozoa are capable of fertilizing an oocyte when taken from the testis
E. human spermatozoa when mature have undergone a reduction division of their nucleus

15. **Regarding miscarriage**

A. if recurrent, it can be associated with uterine malformation
B. if recurrent, it can be associated with sickle cell trait
C. the diagnosis of incomplete miscarriage is assisted by digital examination of the cervical canal
D. cervical incompetence commonly causes recurrent first-trimester miscarriage
E. missed abortion should be suspected if the uterine size is greater than expected for gestational age

16. **Circulatory changes in a healthy woman during a normal pregnancy include**

A. a significant rise in cardiac output only during the second and third trimesters
B. a reduction in tidal volume
C. an increase in glomerular filtration rate
D. a reduction in peripheral blood flow
E. a uterine blood flow at term of the order of 200 ml/minute

17. **Termination of pregnancy**

A. is illegal after 20 weeks gestation
B. after 14 weeks is most safely achieved by hysterotomy
C. requires the signature of a consultant gynaecologist
D. can be achieved by the intra-amniotic administration of prostaglandin
E. complications include infertility in about 10–15% of cases

18. **In ectopic pregnancy**

A. the gestation sac is always within the fallopian tube
B. the diagnosis can be excluded by ultrasound
C. β-HCG levels are detectable in a concentrated urinary sample
D. there may be a coexistent intrauterine pregnancy
E. the patient may present with brown vaginal discharge

19. Hypertension in pregnancy

A. is of no significance unless accompanied by proteinuria
B. causes fetal growth retardation in more than 80% of affected women
C. is associated with an increased incidence of placental praevia
D. must be assessed by admission to hospital for at least 48 hours
E. is a contraindication to the use of intravenous ergometrine

20. In pre-eclampsia

A. the perinatal mortality is raised
B. epigastric pain may indicate impending eclampsia
C. there are lowered serum urate levels
D. there may be no fetus
E. the liquor volume may be diminished

21. A diagnosis of severe dyskaryosis taken on a cervical smear during pregnancy

A. is likely to have been confused with the normal cytological changes of pregnancy
B. is more likely to indicate an adenocarcinoma rather than CIN 3
C. is investigated by colposcopically directed biopsy postnatally
D. is a contraindication to intercourse
E. is an indication for delivery by elective caesarean section

22. Insulin-dependent diabetes mellitus in pregnancy

A. is associated with an increased risk of congenital abnormality
B. reduces maternal insulin requirements
C. is best monitored by urine testing
D. is taken into consideration when interpretating the triple test
E. can be associated with fetal growth retardation

23. Heavy menstrual bleeding can be treated with

A. the combined oral contraceptive pill
B. tranexamic acid, taken during menstruation
C. medicated intrauterine devices
D. danazol, taken during menstruation
E. mefanamic acid, taken days 19 to 26 of the cycle

24. Dysmenorrhoea

A. can be successfully treated with non-steroidal anti-inflammatory drugs
B. can be caused by anovulation
C. is more severe with a retroverted uterus
D. can be caused by endometriosis
E. can be caused by cystocele

25. The progesterone-only pill

A. is liable to cause amenorrhoea
B. can be safely given to lactating women
C. should not be prescribed to an individual with a history of a deep venous thrombosis
D. acts mainly by inhibiting ovulation
E. increases tubal motility

26. The intra-uterine device

A. carries at least a 1 in 4 chance of expulsion
B. may cause menorrhagia
C. increases the risk of miscarriage should pregnancy occur
D. is contraindicated with a past history of ectopic pregnancies
E. significantly increases the risk of fetal abnormality should pregnancy occur

27. Epidurals sited during labour

A. are contraindicated in footling breech deliveries
B. are indicated when a coagulation defect is present
C. lower the maternal blood pressure
D. decrease the rate of rotational forceps deliveries
E. have similar analgesic efficacy to a pudendal nerve block

28. Induction of labour

A. can be achieved by amniotomy
B. is easiest when the cervix is in a posterior position
C. can be achieved by an ergometrine infusion
D. is indicated with an uncomplicated breech presentation of greater than 37 weeks gestation
E. is rarely achieved when vaginal prostin gel is used

29. Delay in the first stage of labour may be caused by

A. a fractured coccyx
B. cephalopelvic disproportion
C. maternal anaemia
D. a brow presentation
E. dehiscence of a caesarean section scar

30. Delay in the second stage of labour may be caused by

A. a rigid perineum
B. a short umbilical cord
C. cervical stenosis following a knife cone biopsy
D. an effective epidural
E. maternal exhaustion

Answers

1.   A – **T**   premature ovarian failure occurs in less than 1% of
women under 40 and has a variety of causes including
genetic, autoimmune, infective, Iatrogenic and
idiopathic

   B – **F**   when ovarian failure occurs there is a *decrease* in HDL

   C – **T**   after ovarian failure there is an additional effect over
and above that of age-related bone loss

   D – **F**   the KPI is the ratio of superficial cells to para basal
cells. Women in the reproductive age group have a
high KPI (estrogenic stimulation gives rise to a higher
number of superficial cells). Prepubertal and
postmenopausal women have a very low KPI

   E – **F**   the average age of menopause in the UK is 50 years 9
months

2.   A – **T**   abnormalities of thyroid function can produce a variety
of menstrual disturbances

   B – **T**   these tumours are rare (<1% of ovarian tumours) and
may present with physical signs of virilization, genital
or breast atrophy as well as menstrual disturbances

   C – **F**   imperforate hymen is associated with *primary*
amenorrhoea

   D – **T**   over-vigorous curettage of the endometrial cavity,
especially in the presence of infection, may cause
scarring and obliteration of the cavity, with subsequent
amenorrhoea

   E – **F**   endometriosis is associated with pelvic pain,
dyspareunia and dysmenorrhoea, not secondary
amenorrhoea

3.   A – **T**   sperm and egg fuse in the fimbrial/ampullary end of
the fallopian tube and transport between this region
and implantation in the endometrium takes between 5
and 7 days

   B – **F**   oophoritis is a very *uncommon* complication of mumps
in the female

   C – **T**   in broad terms infertility can be categorized as being
30% male factor, 30% female factor and 30%

combined factors
D – **T** hyperstimulation is a more common complication when parenteral hormone methods are used to induce ovarian follicles
E – **T** assisted sperm entry into the ovum may overcome the problems of infertility in instances of a markedly reduced sperm count

4. A – **T** it is essential that patients about to undergo male sterilization are made aware that the failure rate is 1 in 300 cases before giving their consent
B – **F** this association has not been confirmed by scientific data
C – **T** anxiety regarding an ectopic pregnancy is often only alleviated when a successful sterilizing procedure is undertaken
D – **F** a number of well-controlled studies have shown that there is no change to the volume of menstrual bleeding experienced by women after tubal ligation
E – **F** success rates vary from surgeon to surgeon, but in general success rates of approximately 50% are quoted. Individual expertise and the use of microsurgical techniques may improve the chances of success

5. A – **T** multiple gestations exacerbate all the complications of pregnancy
B – **F** as heparin does not cross the placenta it therefore does not directly affect the fetus and is not known to have teratogenic effects
C – **T** warfarin crosses the placenta and has been associated with a variety of adverse effects including an increased risk of fetal intra-cerebral and retro-placental haemorrhage
D – **T** long-term therapy of at least 10,000 units per day for 3 months can cause this complication
E – **F** an increased risk is associated with blood groups *other than* O

6.   A – T   in Europe and North America twin births account for 11 per 1000 deliveries; worldwide monozygous twins are present in 3.5 per 1000 births

     B – F   dizygotic twins are familial

     C – F   monozygotic twins can vary from monochorionic and monoamnioic. Dizygotic twins are always dichorionic and diamnioic

     D – T   the increased size of the placenta in monozygotic twins means that there is a greater chance of some part of it encroaching upon the lower segment

     E – T   the incidence of polyhydramnios increases with multiple pregnancy

7.   A – T   open neural tube defect is associated with spina bifida and forms the basis of α-fetoprotein screening in pregnancy

     B – T   although routine ultrasound scans are usually performed in the 2nd trimester spina bifida abnormalities may be diagnosed by ultrasound scans in the 3rd trimester

     C – F   spina bifida does not follow a chromosomal pattern of inheritance

     D – T   characteristic ultrasonic findings in the fetal head are ventriculomegaly, the lemon and banana sign and a reduced BPD (bi-parietal diameter) and head circumferance

     E – T   the triple test involves measurements of maternal serum for unconjugated oestriol, human chorionic gonadotrophin and α-fetoprotein. The latter can therefore be used to screen for open neural tube defects

8.   A – T   presence of Müllerian inhibitory factor is required for the normal development of the Wolffian ducts along the male pattern. In its absence the Müllerian ducts contribute to the female phenotype

     B – T   fetal sexing can be performed ultrasonographically at this stage, but not with 100% diagnostic accuracy

     C – T   normal uterine anatomy results from fusion of portions of the Müllerian ducts from both sides and breakdown

of the midline septum. Failure of this process can
result in a variety of anatomical abnormalities

D – F   the *lower* third of the vagina is formed from the cloaca

E – T   the Wolffian duct persists in the presence of a Y
chromosome

9.   A – F   an XO genotype is associated with *female* somatotype
and is termed Turner's syndrome

      B – F   the total number of chromosomes in both males and
females is *46*

      C – T   this test relies on the presence of inactivate X
chromosome, and can still be seen in males with XXY
composition

      D – F   CVS are associated with a fetal loss in the region of
3% and amniocentesis in the region of 0.5–1%

      E – F   in the presence of a Y chromosome the Müllerian
inhibitory factor suppresses development of the female
genital organs

10. A – F   transitional epithelium lines the urinary tract

      B – F   at the time of ovulation the mucus is typically clear and
profuse

      C – T   the squamo-columnar junction is under hormonal
influence and so alters during puberty and the
menopause

      D – F   non-keratinized stratified epithelium lines the vagina
and encroaches upon the cervix

      E – F   the squamo-columnar junction usually recedes within
the endocervical canal after the menopause

11. A – T   the bi-parietal diameter gradually enlarges during
pregnancy and its ultrasonic measurement assists in
pregnancy dating during the later part of the first and
the second trimester

      B – F   the lambdoidal suture runs between the parietal,
temporal and occipital bones

      C – F   the bregma (also known as the anterior fontanelle) lies
between the frontal and parietal bones

      D – T   the sub-occipito bregmatic diameter presents the

smallest cephalic dimension for passing through the maternal pelvis

E – T   each presentation has a denominator: the chin is the denominator in a face presentation and the sacrum is the denominator in a breech presentation

12. A – T   this is the reverse of the adult situation. Here the arteries carry the de-oxygenated blood

B – F   closure of the ductus arteriosus is a postnatal phenomenon

C – T   primitive placental circulation starts shortly after implantation

D – T   as a part of ultrasonic screening to rule out congenital anomalies, visualization of a 4-chamber heart excludes a number of the major cardiac malformations

E – T   ideally forward flow should occur in both systole and diastole during doppler flow studies of the umbilical arteries

13. A – T   the posterior lobe of the human pituitary gland secretes oxytocin and vasopressin (ADH)

B – F   thyroid stimulation hormone is secreted from the *anterior* lobe

C – F   luteinizing hormone is secreted from the *anterior* lobe

D – F   adrenocorticotrophin is secreted from the *anterior* lobe

E – F   prolactin is secreted from the *anterior* lobe

14. A – F   the vast majority of ejaculate is composed of secretions added from the various glands in the male reproductive tract – from the seminal vesicles, the prostate, the bulbourethral and urethral glands

B – F   the fertilized ovum implants days after fertilization, well past the 16-cell stage

C – F   there is a 'window' of about 24 hours during which the ovum can be fertilized

D – T   direct semen injection into the human oocyte and fertilization has been achieved, following sperm harvesting from the testis

E – T   human spermatozoa carry 23 chromosomes

15. A – **T**   there is an association between miscarriage or
pre-term labour and structural uterine abnormality

B – **F**   recurrent miscarriage is associated with sickle cell
disease, not trait

C – **T**   the internal cervical os is open with an incomplete
miscarriage

D – **F**   cervical incompetence is commonly associated with
second trimester recurrent miscarriage

E – **F**   the uterus is more commonly *smaller* than would be
expected for gestational age

16. A – **F**   the cardiac output rises in the *first* trimester and
continues to rise in the second and third, reaching a
plateau in the third trimester

B – **F**   tidal volume *increases*

C – **T**   glomerular filtration rate (GFR) increases by 55% in
early pregnancy and up to 60% in late pregnancy

D – **F**   peripheral blood flow *increases* and is associated with a
fall in peripheral vascular resistance

E – **F**   uterine blood flow at term is approximately *500*
ml/minute

17. A – **F**   termination of pregnancy for social reasons has an
upper gestation limit of 24 weeks; however in the
presence of fetal abnormality no such upper limit
exists

B – **F**   hysterotomy is rarely used to achieve termination of
pregnancy; prostaglandin induction of uterine
contractions is a safe and successful method

C – **F**   termination of pregnancy requires the signature of *two*
independent medical practitioners

D – **T**   prostaglandin can be given by the vaginal,
extra-amniotic, intra-amniotic and intravenous routes

E – **F**   infertility is a rare complication in termination of
pregnancy

18. A – **F**   the definition of an ectopic pregnancy is conception
outside the uterine cavity not specifically within the
fallopian tube. Other sites include abdominal, cervical

and ovarian pregnancies

B – F   although ultrasound, particularly by the vaginal route, has increased the ability to identify an ectopic pregnancy, the diagnosis is still commonly made on clinical grounds

C – T   sensitive β-HCG urine tests are nearly always positive in the presence of any pregnancy, including those that are ectopic

D – T   the incidence of heterotropic pregnancy in the uterine cavity coexisting with another pregnancy elsewhere is in the region of 1 in 30,000

E – T   some vaginal bleeding, which could be a small quantity of brown discharge or moderate fresh blood, may be present with an ectopic pregnancy

19. A – F   although hypertension in pregnancy can be classified by the presence or absence of proteinuria, events such as cerebrovascular accidents can occur with an elevated blood pressure unaccompanied by proteinuria

B – F   patients with hypertension, medically treated or not, are usually screened to detect fetal growth retardation by serial ultrasound measurement. The majority will have only mild to moderate disease, which may not be associated with fetal growth outside the normal range

C – F   hypertension is associated with an increased incidence of placental abruption

D – F   many cases of hypertension can be successfully managed on an outpatient basis

E – T   ergometrine, given intravenously or intramuscularly postpartum in combination with oxytocin, should be withheld. Oxytocin alone is preferred

20. A – T   perinatal mortality is increased due to a variety of factors, the necessity for preterm delivery being one of the most significant

B – T   epigastric pain, visual disturbances, hyper-reflexia and clonus are all signs of impending eclampsia

C – F   serum urate levels tend to be *elevated* in pre-eclampsia

D – T   pre-eclampsia can occur without a fetus with a hydatidiform mole

E – **T**   poor placental perfusion and diminished fetal renal perfusion can result in a reduction in liquor production

21. A – **F**   pregnancy does not cause dyskaryotic cell appearances and therefore there is no reason to deny cervical screening during pregnancy

B – **F**   severe dyskaryosis is more likely to be associated with the histological diagnosis of CIN 3. Adenocarcinoma is associated with glandular cell abnormality and is far less likely

C – **F**   a diagnosis of severe dyskaryosis in pregnancy is an indication for an urgent colposcopy assessment by an experienced operator to rule out invasive disease

D – **F**   sexual intercourse has not been shown to have any influence on the progression of severe dyskaryosis

E – **F**   vaginal delivery can be safely and successfully achieved in the presence of severe dyskaryosis

22. A – **T**   a variety of congenital abnormalities are associated with diabetes mellitus; most studies have documented a 2- to 4-fold increase

B – **F**   maternal insulin requirements *increase* progressively during the course of pregnancy

C – **F**   urine testing for glycosuria is notoriously inaccurate, and capillary or venous blood samples are essential for monitoring control

D – **T**   women with insulin-dependent diabetes mellitus have significantly lower maternal α-fetoprotein and unconjugated oestriol levels, when compared with women without diabetes. This information is therefore needed to prevent an excess of false positive triple test results in diabetic women

E – **T**   severe diabetics can have poor placental perfusion resulting in fetal growth retardation

23. A – **T**   the combined oral contraceptive pill reduces menstrual blood loss by an average of 50%

B – **T**   the antifibrinolytic tranexamic acid is taken for the duration of the menses and is associated with a reduction of blood loss in the region of 50%

C – **T**   intrauterine devices which release small quantities of either antifibrinolytic or progestagen have been shown to reduce menstrual blood loss

D – **F**   danazol must be taken on a daily basis to influence menstrual blood loss

E – **F**   mefanamic acid is taken during the time of the period

24.   A – **T**   non-steroidal anti-inflammatory drugs have been shown to be effective in reducing dysmenorrhoea, possibly by reducing prostaglandin-induced uterine contractions

B – **F**   ovulatory menstrual cycles are typically associated with spasmodic dysmenorrhoea

C – **F**   a retroverted uterus, not associated with pelvic pathology, is not responsible for an increased severity of dysmenorrhoea

D – **T**   dysmenorrhoea can be a prominent feature of women suffering from endometriosis

E – **F**   cystocele is not associated with menstrually-related discomfort or pain

25.   A – **T**   taking the progesterone-only pill may be associated with either regular menstrual cycles, erratic vaginal bleeding or amenorrhoea

B – **T**   the *combined* oral contraceptive pill is not advised during lactation

C – **F**   there is no association between the progesterone-only pill and thrombo-embolic disease

D – **F**   only 40% of women taking the progesterone-only pill have their ovulation inhibited; the POP's main action is in thickening the cervical mucus

E – **F**   the progesterone-only pill *decreases* tubal motility hence its association with tubal ectopic pregnancy

26.   A – **F**   expulsion of an intrauterine device is more common in nulliparous women compared with parous women Expulsions vary between 1 and 10 per 100 women in the first year of use

B – **T**   the inert intrauterine contraceptive device has been shown to increase menstrual loss and therefore the incidence of menorrhagia

C – **T**   removal of an intrauterine contraceptive device in early pregnancy is warranted despite the risk of miscarriage, as the miscarriage risk is even greater if the device is left *in situ*

D – **T**   intrauterine contraceptive devices only prevent intrauterine pregnancies

E – **F**   an intrauterine contraceptive device increases the risk of miscarriage, not fetal abnormality

27.   A – **F**   epidurals are commonly recommended for all types of breech presentation

B – **F**   the siting of an epidural is contraindicated in the presence of a coagulopathy because of the risk of bleeding from the venous sinuses

C – **T**   an epidural causes peripheral dilation and pooling of the blood thereby lowering the maternal blood pressure

D – **F**   epidurals are associated with an *increased* rate of rotational forceps deliveries owing to a loss of tone in the pelvic musculature

E – **F**   the analgesic effect of a pudendal nerve block is limited to the nerve distribution of sacral nerves two, three and four

28.   A – **T**   amniotomy, which may need to be followed by an oxytocin infusion, is a successful means of inducing labour

B – **F**   the cervix is *least* favourable when in the posterior position. Anterior is best

C – **F**   ergometrine causes tonic contraction of the uterus and is therefore inappropriate for the induction of labour

D – **F**   the highest chance of a successful vaginal delivery with a breech presentation is with the spontaneous onset of labour. Therefore, routine induction of labour cannot be justified

E – **F**   induction of labour using vaginal prostin gel has a high incidence of success

29. A – F   the first stage of labour requires the cervix to become fully dilated and is reliant upon adequate uterine activity. It is not restricted by the bony pelvis

     B – T   if inefficient uterine activity has been excluded, delay in the later part of the first stage of labour may be suggestive of cephalopelvic disproportion

     C – F   maternal anaemia is not associated with delay in any stage of labour

     D – T   with the exception of the pre-term fetus, a brow presentation is not normally deliverable vaginally and is an important presentation to exclude when delay in the first stage is noted

     E – T   cessation of previously good progress in labour of a woman who has had a previous Caesarean section should alert the clinician to the possibility of scar dehiscence

30. A – T   an episiotomy can overcome the problem of a rigid perineum delaying the second stage of labour

     B – F   the length of the umbilical cord varies greatly but in practice never prevents delivery

     C – F   the diagnosis of the second stage of labour cannot be made until full cervical dilatation has been achieved

     D – T   the lack of expulsive sensation in the presence of an adequately working epidural can cause the second stage to be prolonged

     E – T   maternal exhaustion, which can be multifactorial, is a common cause of delay in the second stage

MCQs: Paper 2

1. **Down's syndrome**

A. has a birth prevalence in the region of 1.4 per 1000 in England and Wales
B. can be diagnosed using the triple test
C. can be found in mosaic form
D. is associated with oligohydramnios
E. is associated with a higher rate of miscarriage than in pregnancies with a normal karyotype

2. **Concerning post-coital contraception**

A. the progesterone only pill (POP) has a role
B. oral methods should be administered within 24 hours
C. is available as an 'over the counter' preparation
D. the intrauterine device has a role
E. requires no follow-up visit

3. **Urinary tract infection in pregnancy**

A. is associated with pre-term labour
B. is commonly due to staphylococci
C. acute pyelonephritis is associated with intrauterine growth retardation
D. is more common with a transverse lie
E. may present with vomiting

4. Rubella in pregnancy

A. screening for immunity should be discussed with every pregnant woman when first seen in the antenatal clinic and sampling for rubella antibodies advised
B. is associated with recurrent miscarriage
C. is associated with the greatest incidence of congenital malformations when the infection occurs during the second trimester
D. is indicated by a rising titre of rubella-specific IgM levels following recent infection
E. is associated with a neural tube defect in the fetus

5. Congenital fetal malformations are associated with the following maternal infections

A. hepatitis B
B. toxoplasmosis
C. cytomegalovirus
D. measles
E. parvovirus

6. Concerning thalassaemia in pregnancy

A. thalassaemia minor may be suspected on a blood film
B. it most commonly occurs in women of African origin
C. the carrier rate in the UK is approximately 1 in 10,000
D. a woman with β-thalassaemia minor can be reassured that the baby will be healthy
E. thalassaemia trait increases the likelihood of pre-eclampsia

7. LHRH analogues

A. can be used to treat endometriosis
B. rarely cause side-effects
C. can be administered orally
D. are inexpensive preparations
E. act principally at the uterine level

8. Concerning intermenstrual bleeding (IMB)

A. IMB occurs in about 10% of normal menstrual cycles
B. laparoscopy should be included as part of the investigation
C. a luteal phase progesterone is essential
D. IMB may be associated with ovulation
E. IMB is a feature of cervical intra-epithelial neoplasia

9. Risks of combined oral contraceptive (COC) pill usage include

A. increased incidence of endometrial carcinoma
B. pelvic inflammatory disease
C. benign ovarian cysts
D. hypotension
E. increased risk of ovarian carcinoma

10. Rotational delivery

A. may be preceded with a labour during which back pain is a prominent feature
B. can be achieved using a Silastic ventouse cup
C. can be safely attempted when two-fifths of the fetal head are palpable per abdomen
D. can correct a deep transverse arrest
E. should be attempted with a fetal pH of 7.12

11. In pregnancy, ultrasound

A. can diagnose fetal ascites
B. anomaly scanning is usually carried out in the second trimester of pregnancy
C. can establish fetal maturity at 34 weeks gestation
D. can diagnose a cleft lip
E. is able to identify the fertilized ovum, prior to implantation

12. The following are known to be teratogenic

A. alcohol
B. methyldopa
C. warfarin
D. aminoglycosides
E. phenytoin

13. Fallopian tube occlusion

A. may be caused by chlamydial infection
B. is a common finding in pelvic endometriosis
C. when caused by infection most commonly ascends from the lower genital tract
D. may follow appendicitis
E. can be assessed using transvaginal ultrasound

14. Gonorrhoea

A. may cause blindness in the baby of an infected mother
B. is diagnosed by taking a high vaginal swab
C. may cause perihepatitis
D. may cause penile discharge
E. is caused by a Gram-positive diplococcus

15. The following instructions are appropriate when advising on the use of the diaphragm

A. always use a spermicide
B. sterilize the diaphragm prior to insertion
C. the diaphragm cannot be used at the same time as the sheath
D. refitting of the diaphragm is required after childbirth
E. the diaphragm must be left in place for at least 6 hours following intercourse

16. Concerning sickle cell disorders in pregnancy

A. sickle cell disorders are most common in women of Asian origin
B. a sickle cell crisis can be precipitated in conditions of heightened oxygen tension
C. sickle cell disorders are associated with an increased incidence of hypertension during pregnancy
D. sickle cell disease results from a variant on the alpha globin chain
E. partner screening is recommended during the second trimester

17. Urodynamic investigations

A. are unnecessary in the patient who complains of stress incontinence
B. can be conducted before excluding urinary infection
C. cystometry measures the pressure/volume relationship of the bladder during filling and voiding
D. could usefully include ultrasonography
E. if normal, should show a bladder capacity of 250 ml

18. The perinatal mortality rate

A. is usually expressed as the rate per thousand total births over 1 year
B. is attributable to congenital malformations in 50% of cases
C. in England and Wales is higher in those whose mother was born in Pakistan than those whose mother was born in the West Indies
D. falls with social class
E. is lowest in mothers aged between 18 and 20 years

19. Tocolysis to suppress pre-term labour

A. ideally should be continued for 12 hours
B. carries the risk of maternal pulmonary oedema
C. is usually initiated with oral therapy
D. may be employed beyond 34 weeks gestation
E. is exclusively a role for β-sympathomimetics

20. Ovarian masses

A. are malignant in the presence of ascites
B. include benign teratomas
C. of germ cell origin may secrete hormones
D. may be confused with developmental abnormalities of the renal tract
E. if malignant can be reliably staged pre-operatively

21. Concerning lactation

A. lactation is successfully suppressed by demand feeding to empty the engorged breasts
B. colostrum is secreted for seven days after the birth
C. bromocryptine promotes milk production
D. lactation will fall in Sheehan's syndrome
E. the staphylococcus organism is associated with puerperal mastitis

22. When massive post-partum haemorrhage occurs

A. an anaesthetist is essential to assist in the management of the patient
B. initial cross-matching of 3 units of blood is sufficient
C. bimanual uterine compression has a role
D. uncross-matched O rhesus-positive blood may be given in an emergency
E. bilateral uterine artery ligation may be necessary

23. Secondary post-partum haemorrhage

A. is abnormal bleeding that occurs 12 hours post-partum
B. may be due to infection
C. cannot be controlled by uterine contracting agents
D. occurs following 5% of births
E. can usually be diagnosed by ultrasound examination of the pelvic organs

24. Regarding resuscitation of the newborn

A. resuscitation in some form is required by approximately one-third of babies
B. the Apgar score is recorded at delivery
C. resuscitation will be required if the fetal heart rate is persistently 90 beats a minute
D. meconium seen in the posterior pharynx and larynx is an indication for intubation
E. naloxone can be given safely to all infants

25. Concerning maternal cardiac disease in pregnancy

A. a classification system exists to determine the mortality risk
B. involvement of the aorta in Marfan's syndrome increases the mortality
C. the fetus has an increased risk of congenital heart disease
D. mitral stenosis is an infrequent complication following rheumatic heart disease
E. women with primary pulmonary hypertension should be advised against pregnancy

26. Appropriate investigations of a term stillbirth would include

A. maternal glycosylated haemoglobin
B. a Kleihauer blood test
C. a platelet count
D. blood pressure measurement
E. antinuclear antibody estimation

27. Fetal antenatal surveillance using the biophysical profile

A. includes an assessment of fetal breathing
B. has a score with a maximum value of 12
C. includes an assessment of fetal heart rate reactivity
D. does not take note of amniotic fluid volume
E. includes an assessment of fetal tone and posture

28. Placental abruption

A. may have no associated vaginal bleeding
B. is an indication for delivery
C. has a higher incidence with maternal cocaine abuse
D. may be identified using ultrasound by demonstrating retroplacental clot
E. can be readily distinguished from acute appendicitis

29. The ventouse method

A. may employ a metal cup
B. has increased in popularity with electronic pumps
C. can be used safely in the absence of criteria necessary for a forceps delivery
D. requires the patient to be in the lithotomy position
E. may be performed in conjunction with a pudendal block

30. A high fetal head at term in a primipara

A. can be caused by placenta praevia
B. can be caused by a lower segment uterine fibroid
C. is associated with incorrect pregnancy dating
D. is an indication for a Caesarean section
E. has a higher incidence in patients of African origin

Answers

1. A – **T**   this figure translates into approximately 970 affected
births annually

B – **F**   the triple test only gives a risk for the likely incidence
of Down's syndrome being present at term, in an
individual pregnancy. Diagnosis requires karyotyping

C – **T**   mosaicism accounts for 1–2% of Down's cases

D – **F**   polyhydramnios is found, in association with duodenal
atresia

E – **T**   fetal wastage is more common with all types of
chromosomal abnormalities

2. A – **F**   the POP is not used in this context as its principle
mechanism of action is thickening of cervical mucus
and prevention of sperm penetration

B – **F**   the combination of oestrogen and progesterone
(Yuzpe) method should be administered within 72
hours

C – **F**   a prescription is required

D – **T**   following adequate counselling the intrauterine
contraceptive device may be fitted within 5 days of the
episode of unprotected intercourse

E – **F**   follow-up is necessary to detect the method failures
(approximately 10%), and to ensure adequate
contraceptive measures are being taken

3. A – **T**   uterine activity can be precipitated by urinary infection
and should always be screened for and treated in the
patient who presents with symptoms and/or signs of
pre-term labour

B – **F**   this organism is unusual, the most common bacterium
found is *Escherichia coli*

C – **T**   this association, together with the risks of pre-term
labour and delivery, are the indication for
hospitalization and intravenous antibiotic therapy to
treat acute pyelonephritis

D – **F**   there is no known, statistically proven, association with
fetal lie

E – **T**   a variety of non-specific symptoms may be present,
such as nausea, vomiting, fever and abdominal pain

4.　A – **T**　such screening provides valuable baseline information. Additionally, all women who lack rubella antibodies should be identified and offered post-natal vaccination

　　　B – **F**　a pregnancy during which primary rubella infection is contracted has a higher incidence of miscarriage. Thereafter rubella immunity is developed and protects a subsequent pregnancy from this complication

　　　C – **F**　first-trimester infection has the most devastating consequences, with in excess of 80% of fetuses affected

　　　D – **T**　detection of rising IgM titres is used for diagnostic purposes. Rubella-specific IgM is demonstrable for up to 8 weeks after the onset of the rash

　　　E – **F**　a variety of defects including cataracts, chorioretinitis, micropthalmia, glaucoma, deafness, microcephaly and mental retardation but not neural tube defects are associated with congenital rubella infection

5.　A – **F**　there is no known association. However, infants born to hepatitis B surface-antigen-positive women should be given hepatitis B immunoglobulin and active immunization shortly after delivery

　　　B – **T**　toxoplasmosis infection is associated with fetal intracranial calcification, microcephaly, hydrocephaly and hepatosplenomegaly

　　　C – **T**　cytomegalovirus can result in hepatosplenomegaly, microcephaly, hyperbilirubinaemia, petechiae and thrombocytopenia

　　　D – **F**　measles during pregnancy is not generally associated with an increased fetal death rate, although placental damage from the infection has been implicated in stillbirths

　　　E – **T**　parvovirus B19 infection is a known cause of non-immune hydrops fetalis

6.　A – **T**　red blood cells of sufferers are small with a low mean cell volume and low mean cell haemoglobin

　　　B – **F**　thalassaemia has a worldwide distribution, but is concentrated in a broad band encompassing the Mediterranean and Middle East

　　　C – **T**　the carrier rate of approximately 1 in 10,000 in the UK can be compared with a carrier rate of 1 in 7 in Cyprus

D – F   depending on the carrier status of the mother's partner, the fetus may have a normal haemoglobin, thalassaemia minor or thalassaemia major. Therefore, no such reassurance can be given

E – F   there is no known association

7. A – T   LHRH analogues have proved to be successful therapy for endometriosis in a number of controlled trials

B – F   side-effects, similar to those experienced by women during the menopause, are commonly experienced by women in receipt of LHRH analogue treatment

C – F   the polypeptide structure of the LHRH analogues makes them inappropriate for oral administration. Parenteral routes, including the nasal route, injection and depot preparations have been developed

D – F   costs of these preparations are in excess of £80 per month

E – F   LHRH analogues act by initial stimulation, followed by down-regulation of pituitary gonadotrophin secretion

8. A – F   IMB is uncommon in the normal menstrual cycle

B – F   *hysteroscopy* is the more useful investigation

C – F   the establishment of ovulation is not essential in the management of patients with IMB, but may be helpful if progestagens are to be considered in the adequately assessed anovulatory patient

D – T   regular mid-cycle spotting and pain ('mittelschmerz') are noted by some women at the time of ovulation

E – F   pre-invasive cervical disease does not cause bleeding

9. A – F   the COC has a protective effect in the order of 50%

B – F   the incidence of PID is *lower* in women who use the COC as a method of contraception, compared with women who have unprotected intercourse

C – F   the incidence of benign ovarian cysts is *lower*

D – F   COC usage is associated with *hypertension*

E – F   the COC has a protective effect, most studies indicate a reduction in excess of 50%

10. A – **T** back pain is common in labours with an occipito-posterior position of the fetal head

B – **T** the ventouse has increased in popularity for achieving safe rotational vaginal delivery. Clinicians often prefer the metal cup for rotations, feeling the failure rate is lower

C – **F** none of the head should be palpable per abdomen

D – **T** rotation to the occipito-anterior position can permit vaginal delivery

E – **F** in the presence of fetal distress, delivery should be by Caesarean section

11. A – **T** fluid can clearly be seen around the fetal liver and bowel

B – **T** most commonly this examination is now conducted between the 18th and 20th weeks of gestational age

C – **F** fetal maturity cannot be reliably determined ultrasonographically in the third trimester

D – **T** early diagnosis of cleft lip can be useful information to forewarn the parents and paediatric surgeons

E – **F** pregnancies can only be detected following implantation

12. A – **T** widespread abnormalities, including those of the fetal alcohol syndrome with growth retardation, central nervous system abnormalities, microcephaly, microphthalmia and poorly developed philtrum have been described

B – **F** methyldopa has been used safely during pregnancy for many years to control hypertension. There have been occasional case reports of microcephaly

C – **T** warfarin is known to cause intracerebral haemorrhage, nasal hypoplasia and stippling of the epiphyses

D – **T** aminoglycosides are known to be ototoxic

E – **T** various craniofacial and digital abnormalities, together with more major anomalies have been associated with maternal phenytoin ingestion during pregnancy

13.   A – **T**   chlamydial infection, which may be asymptomatic, can cause considerable tube damage. It is more common than gonorrhoea as the infection responsible

      B – **F**   tubal occlusion is surprisingly uncommon even in the presence of moderately severe pelvic endometriosis

      C – **T**   the mechanism, however, by which infection ascends through the cervical canal and reaches the fallopian tubes is still unknown

      D – **T**   appendicitis can result in tubal damage, both from the local pelvic inflammatory reaction and the associated surgery

      E – **F**   a hydrosalpinx may be seen ultrasonographically, but occlusion of normal calibre tube and fimbrial end clubbing cannot be diagnosed by this means

14.   A – **T**   gonococcal ophthalmia neonatorum can lead to severe conjunctivitis, keratitis and blindness if not promptly treated

      B – **F**   endocervical and urethral swabs are required. In some circumstances throat and rectal swabs should be considered

      C – **T**   systemic manifestations, perihepatitis and septicaemia can all be caused by gonococcal infection

      D – **T**   the majority of gonococcal infected men develop a urethritis, dysuria and urethral discharge

      E – **F**   gonococcus is a Gram-*negative* intracellular diplococcus

15.   A – **T**   the efficacy of the diaphragm as a method of contraception is reduced if this advice is ignored

      B – **F**   the diaphragm should be clean, but sterility is not required

      C – **F**   safer sexual practices are to be encouraged and there is no reason why two barrier methods should not be used together

      D – **T**   it is important to advise re-fitting after each child is born and when there has been a significant weight change in the user

      E – **T**   removal before 6 hours has elapsed following intercourse diminishes the efficacy of the diaphragm method of contraception. If further intercourse takes place before this time, the spermicide should be replenished

16.
A – F   African and West Indian populations have the highest incidence

B – F   *lowered* oxygen tension, acidosis, infection and dehydration may precipitate a crisis

C – T   regular screening for hypertension/pre-eclampsia, urinary tract infection and reduced fetal growth is recommended in women with sickle cell disease

D – F   sickle cell disease results from an amino acid substitution of glutamine for valine on the *beta* globin chain

E – F   earlier (pre-pregnancy or first trimester) diagnosis is recommended so that the couple can be advised on the possible risk of a serious haemoglobin defect in their offspring and subsequently counselled about the means of diagnosis in the fetus

17.
A – F   studies have shown that a significant proportion of women with stress incontinence have detrusor instability and therefore this investigation is worthwhile to prevent inappropriate intervention

B – F   urinary infection may be responsible for some or even all a patient's symptoms and therefore it should always be excluded before conducting time-consuming and invasive investigations

C – T   cystometry is indicated in the investigation of patients with multiple symptoms, a voiding disorder, previous unsuccessful incontinence surgery or a neuropathic bladder disorder

D – T   ultrasound is a means of assessing postmicturition residual urinary volume and the bladder neck

E – F   capacity (taken as a strong desire to void) should be greater than 400 ml

18.   A – **T**   the perinatal mortality rate is the number of perinatal deaths divided by the total births (born live and still) during the same period

        B – **F**   *20%* of deaths are attributable to congenital malformations

        C – **T**   mothers from Pakistan also have a higher perinatal mortality rate than those from India and Bangladesh

        D – **F**   perinatal mortality *rises* with social class: in 1986 the rate was 7.2 per 1000 births in social classes 1 and 2 compared with 11.4 per 1000 births in social class 5 (England and Wales)

        E – **F**   perinatal mortality is lowest in those mothers aged between 20 and 29 years

19.   A – **F**   labour should be suppressed for *48* hours to gain maximum benefit from the steroids used to enhance fetal lung development

        B – **T**   maternal pulmonary oedema is a particular risk with the β-sympathomimetics and warrants careful attention to the patient's fluid balance

        C – **F**   intravenous therapy is almost universally administered initially, the role of oral tocolysis remaining controversial

        D – **T**   although permitting delivery is the usual management when gestation has reached 34 weeks, tocolysis may temporarily suppress labour, enabling in-utero transfer to a unit with more sophisticated obstetric and neonatal facilities

        E – **F**   magnesium sulphate, indomethacin and nifedipine are some of the alternative pharmacological agents that have been investigated

20.   A – **F**   ascites can occur with benign ovarian tumours and parasitic fibroids. Meig's syndrome describes ascites and pleural effusion in association with a benign ovarian fibroma

        B – **T**   teratomas (also known as dermoids) are most common in young women and are bilateral in about 12% of cases

        C – **T**   both α-fetoprotein and human chorionic

gonadotrophin may be produced

D – **T**   a palpable pelvic kidney can simulate an ovarian mass

E – **F**   careful surgical staging is essential to determine the appropriate subsequent management

21. A – **F**   such measures *promote* milk production. Non-feeding, simple analgesia and a good supportive bra are usually adequate measures

B – **F**   colostrum is secreted for approximately the first two days postpartum; the change to milk occurs on the third and fourth day

C – **F**   bromocryptine inhibits the release of prolactin from the pituitary and is therefore useful for the suppression of lactation

D – **T**   Sheehan's syndrome or necrosis of the anterior pituitary following severe postpartum haemorrhage is now fortunately very rare. If the patient survives, there is a failure of lactation due to the lack of prolactin and manifestations of the other endocrine deficiencies

E – **T**   mastitis is associated with milk stasis, nipple trauma and poor nursing technique. Pathogenic bacteria enter and are most commonly of the staphylococcal type

22. A – **T**   the anaesthetist is an essential member of the team and will normally manage the patient's fluid balance, in addition to inserting central intravenous access lines

B – **F**   a minimum of 6 units of blood should be cross-matched

C – **T**   uterine atony resulting in dramatic bleeding may be controlled by forcibly compressing the uterus between a hand on the abdomen and a hand inserted per-vaginum

D – **F**   uncross-matched O rhesus-*negative* blood can be used unless the patient is known to have anti-C antibodies

E – **T**   uterine haemorrhage that cannot be controlled by local or pharmacological means necessitates surgery. Uterine artery ligation may be sufficient to avoid hysterectomy

23. A – F   secondary post-partum haemorrhage is defined as abnormal bleeding that occurs between 24 hours and 6 weeks post-partum

B – T   endometritis is a common cause

C – F   uterine relaxation and atony can occur in the few days following delivery. It may respond to oxytocin, ergometrine or prostaglandin therapy. The possibility of retained products, however, should be borne in mind

D – F   secondary post-partum haemorrhage occurs after approximately 1% of births

E – F   ultrasonic findings are unhelpful earlier than 10 days post-partum and thereafter it may be difficult to distinguish retained products from blood clot

24. A – T   although some form of resuscitation is required by about a third of babies active resuscitation, such as assisted ventilation, is required by less than 5%

B – F   the Apgar score is recorded at 1, 5 and sometimes 10 minutes after delivery

C – T   recognition of the need for resuscitation should be prompt (in the first minute) if there is no regular respiration, the heart rate is below 100 beats/minute or if the Apgar score remains below 7

D – T   gentle suction should be applied to the endotracheal tube until no further meconium is obtained, changing the tube should it become blocked during the process

E – F   care should be taken in the infant of a mother who is a known opiate addict. Use may precipitate acute withdrawal in the neonate

25. A – T   the New York Heart Association Classification is based on the physical abilities of the mother and is divided into 4 classes. Nearly 90% are in the milder categories of 1 and 2; those with class 3 and 4 account for only 10% of heart disease in pregnancy but account for 85% of cardiac-caused deaths

B – T   involvement of the aorta in Marfan's syndrome increases the mortality from 5–15% to 25–50%

C – T   the fetus has a greater risk of congenital heart disease

when the abnormality is present on the maternal side
rather than the paternal one. There is also an
increased incidence of prematurity and intrauterine
growth retardation

D – F   mitral stenosis is the most frequent rheumatic valvular
disorder (90%)

E – T   primary pulmonary hypertension is associated with
sudden death; the raised cardiac output and decreased
peripheral resistance of normal pregnancy increases
the risk to an unacceptable 50%

26. A – T   maternal glycosylated haemoglobin is required for the
detection of diabetes mellitus as glycaemia control may
have returned to within normal limits post-partum

B – T   a Kleihauer blood test is a stain of maternal blood to
establish the presence of fetal red blood cells and
quantitates the volume of feto-maternal transfusion

C – T   an increasing incidence of consumptive coagulopathy
develops with time following fetal demise and
therefore should be checked in a woman with a
retained dead fetus *in utero*

D – T   hypertensive disease of all aetiologies increases
perinatal mortality

E – T   systemic lupus erythematosus is associated with an
increased pregnancy loss in all trimesters

27. A – T   normal behaviour is considered to be one breathing
episode of 30 seconds duration. Continuous, repetitive
or absent breathing is abnormal

B – F   the maximum score is 10

C – T   a cardiotocogram is part of the assessment to make the
biophysical profile score

D – F   a reduction in amniotic fluid volume either by a
reduced depth measurement or a subjective
diminution is considered abnormal

E – T   low-velocity movements, flaccidity and abnormal
position together with the complete absence of fetal
movement are all considered abnormal

28. A – **T**   so called 'concealed' abruptions constitute 20–35% of cases

B – **F**   in cases of mild abruption, particularly with the preterm fetus, provided the fetal condition is monitored, expectant management should be considered

C – **T**   maternal cocaine abuse is associated with a higher incidence of placental abruption and increased risks of growth retardation and preterm labour

D – **T**   the diagnosis of placental abruption is principally a clinical one, but in the presence of a large clot it may be identified as a hyperechogenic area on ultrasound examination

E – **F**   the diagnosis of appendicitis in pregnancy is notoriously difficult and can be confused with concealed placental abruption

29. A – **T**   pliable Silastic cups are increasing in popularity and replacing the metal cups as they are simpler to assemble

B – **T**   electronic pumps produce a rapid onset and reliably controlled vacuum and are therefore preferred to the hand pump devices

C – **F**   the criteria for the ventouse method and forceps should be the same. The role of the ventouse to expedite delivery at less than full dilatation is most controversial

D – **T**   the patient should be in the lithotomy position, similar to a forceps delivery

E – **T**   a pudendal block may be adequate with perineal infiltration of local anaesthetic for the lift out procedures

30. A – **T**   a placenta which significantly encroaches into the lower segment prevents engagement of the fetal head

B – **T**   any 'tumour' which obstructs the lower segment can prevent descent of the fetal head

C – **T**   the preterm infant would not be expected to have engaged in the pelvis and therefore the dating of the pregnancy should be checked. The widespread use of earlier ultrasound has assisted in the more accurate assessment of pregnancy gestation

D – F   significant numbers will experience descent of the head into the pelvis during labour and successful vaginal delivery and therefore routine Caesarean section cannot be justified. The possibility of cephalopelvic disproportion should, however, be borne in mind

E – T   African races commonly have a pelvic inlet with a higher angle of inclination than Caucasian women and therefore the head may fail to engage before the onset of labour

MCQs: Paper 3

1. **Concerning infections of the genital tract**

A. vaginal candidiasis predisposes to oral infections of the neonate
B. *Gardnerella vaginalis* is encouraged by an increase in the number of döderleins bacilli in the vagina
C. vaginal discharge due to *Candida albicans* is effectively treated by metronidazole
D. metronidazole is contraindicated in late pregnancy
E. gonorrhoea causes bartholinitis

2. **Cervical polyps**

A. cause spontaneous abortion
B. are a cause of antepartum haemorrhage
C. cause watery vaginal discharge
D. are covered by sqaumous epithelium
E. cause intermenstrual bleeding

3. **Regarding female micturition**

A. retention of urine may be due to an enterocoele
B. urge incontinence associated with detrusor instability is improved by pelvic floor exercises
C. detrusor instability is associated with upper motor neurone lesions
D. if a woman presents with mainly stress incontinence, urodynamics are not needed
E. acute retention may be due to haematocolpos

4. Prolapse

A. may prevent complete emptying of the bladder
B. is more common in women of African origin
C. if second degree may be treated by a Hodge pessary
D. is associated with a large uterus
E. occurs only after the menopause

5. Transverse lie

A. is associated with a double uterus
B. is associated with multiple pregnancy
C. is the commonest lie of the second twin
D. can be found with an antepartum haemorrhage
E. should be delivered by classical Caesarean section

6. Regarding the maternal mortality report for the years 1988–1990

A. substandard care was implicated in nearly 25% of deaths
B. the main causes of direct maternal deaths were cerebral hypertensive disorders and haemorrhage
C. the number of maternal deaths due to haemorrhage had doubled since the previous triennium
D. deaths due to anaesthesia had decreased
E. the direct obstetric mortality rate was higher in England than in Northern Ireland

7. Regarding carcinoma of the endometrium

A. risk factors include opposed HRT
B. it can be diagnosed by an endometrial biopsy
C. common UK treatment is a radical hysterectomy followed by external beam radiotherapy
D. the incidence is lower in thin women as they have more conversion of androgen precursors to oestrone
E. can be preceded by cystic or adenomatous hyperplasia

8. Regarding uterine inversion

A. it should not occur if the third stage of labour is managed appropriately
B. it should prompt suspicion of morbid adherence of the placenta
C. if the placenta is attached it should be removed immediately
D. it can be replaced by the hydrostatic method
E. the uterus should not be replaced before anaesthesia (GA, epidural or spinal) is administered

9. Concerning the vulva

A. unilateral enlargement can be due to a hydrocoele of the canal of Gordon
B. pruritus vulvae can be caused by pox virus
C. with atrophic dystrophies testosterone cream may be useful
D. vulval carcinoma forms about 10% of all female genital tract cancers
E. vulval carcinoma may present with the symptoms of intractable pruritus

10. A woman presents with a history of 7 weeks amenorrhoea followed by 6 weeks of mild vaginal bleeding

A. she may have a tubal pregnancy
B. if the urinary pregnancy test is negative an ectopic is excluded
C. she may be miscarrying
D. she may have inadequate luteal phase
E. if she has dysfunctional uterine bleeding high-dose progestagens should stop the bleeding

11. Regarding neonatal medicine

A. all normal term babies lose weight after delivery but regain their birthweight by 5 days
B. neonates with phenylketonuria should not be breastfed
C. erythema toxicum has a high mortality
D. jaundice occurring in the first 24 hours is most likely to be physiological and is due to increased unconjugated bilirubin levels
E. excessive oxygen administration in the preterm infant can cause retinopathy

12. Regarding male fertility

A. azoospermia may respond to steroid treatment
B. in a semen sample 5 white blood cells (WBCs) per high-power field is normal
C. in a semen sample 40% of abnormal forms is acceptable
D. low FSH and LH suggest testicular failure
E. micromanipulation of the zona pellucida increases fertility rates

13. Laparoscopies

A. have a mortality rate of approximately 1 in 30,000
B. may be complicated by an H_2O embolus
C. commonly produce shoulder-tip pain postoperatively
D. should always be preceded by emptying of the bladder
E. can cause peritonitis

14. Regarding hydatidiform mole

A. the incidence is higher in Indonesia than Australia
B. the uterus may be smaller than the dates signify
C. it may present with symptoms and signs of pre-eclampsia
D. it must be followed up by the local hospital
E. a subsequent pregnancy can stimulate a recurrence

15. A woman suddenly collapses 5 minutes after a normal delivery

A. the first priorities are to insert an IV line, then establish an airway, then ventilate
B. if she has had an amniotic fluid embolism she may develop disseminated intravascular coagulopathy (DIC)
C. she is having a massive postpartum haemorrhage so the most likely cause is a tear of the cervical artery
D. she has had a previous Caesarean section, but as she has just had a normal delivery, uterine rupture could not be a cause
E. a pulmonary embolus is unlikely as she has had a normal delivery

16. The following conditions cause ambiguous external genitalia in the neonate

A. Turner's syndrome
B. testicular feminization (androgen insensitivity)
C. cryptorchidism
D. adrenogenital syndrome
E. Klinefelter's syndrome

17. The following changes occur in the mother during normal pregnancy

A. the blood urea level falls to 3.0 mmol/L or less
B. there is a decrease in mucoid discharge from the cervix
C. respiratory tidal volume falls
D. there is an increase in cardiac output by 8 weeks gestation
E. fasting blood glucose levels in the first trimester are greater than in the non-pregnant state

18. In severe eclampsia

A. the creatinine clearance rate is higher than in normal pregnancy
B. there are defects of the development of the placental bed in the second trimester
C. there is an increased incidence of placental abruption
D. the intravascular compartment is increased
E. plasma urea levels are raised

19. Regarding rhesus disease

A.   anti-D should be given if antibodies are detected in early pregnancy
B.   it may be caused by genetic amniocentesis
C.   rhesus disease is routinely prevented by giving anti-D gammaglobulin in the first trimester of pregnancy
D.   is not present if the Kleihauer test is negative
E.   is more likely to occur in a rhesus-negative mother with an ABO-incompatible fetus

20. The fetal head is said to be engaged when

A.   it becomes fixed in the pelvic brim
B.   the leading part is 1 cm above the ischial spines
C.   the biparietal diameter has passed through the pelvic brim
D.   one fifth of the fetal head is palpable abdominally
E.   the caput succedaneum reaches the level of the ischial spines

21. Ovulation in the human is

A.   accompanied by a surge of follicle-stimulating hormone
B.   characteristically followed by the development of secretory endometrium
C.   followed by increased ferning of the cervical mucus
D.   associated with a sustained rise in basal body temperature
E.   occurs 14 days before the next menstrual period

22. With regard to HRT in the postmenopausal woman

A.   with a history of thromboembolic disease oral therapy is preferable to transdermal
B.   premarin 0.625 mg is adequate for prevention of bone loss
C.   cystic hyperplasia must be treated by Wertheims hysterectomy
D.   an endometrial thickness of 3 mm suggests hyperplasia
E.   oestrogen replacement therapy will decrease HDL levels

23. In vaginal breech delivery

A. delay in the second stage is usually treated by oxytocin
B. it is best managed by extraction soon after full cervical dilatation
C. when the legs are extended the presenting diameter is the ditrochanteric
D. the commonest cause of perinatal death is prematurity
E. the fetal back (sacrum) should be kept posterior

24. Regarding maternal mortality in the UK

A. the maternal mortality rate 1988–1990 was 10 per 10,000 births
B. deaths related to hypertension are most commonly caused by cardiac failure
C. emergency general anaesthesia contributes to death from Mendelssohn's syndrome
D. the number of deaths from pulmonary embolism after Caesarean section has not fallen during the past 20 years
E. in modern obstetrics amniotic fluid embolism should be preventable

25. Hyperprolactinaemia

A. is a cause of infertility in women
B. may be treated with dopamine antagonist drugs
C. may be difficult to diagnose with certainty
D. can by physiological
E. is caused by an adenoma of the posterior pituitary gland

26. The premenstrual syndrome (PMS)

A. has a low placebo response rate
B. may respond to dietary manipulation
C. diagnosis must be supported by written or visual evidence
D. can be treated by ovulation suppression
E. does not respond to mefenamic acid

27. Regarding syphilis

A. palmar rash is a sign of secondary syphilis
B. the primary chancre heals spontaneously after 5–8 days
C. presenting signs are often condylomata acuminata
D. the regional lymph nodes become enlarged, soft and very tender in primary disease
E. secondary syphilis has a low infectivity

28. Carcinoma of the cervix

A. classically presents with postmenopausal bleeding
B. if stage 1b it can be treated with a Wertheim's hysterectomy and conservation of the ovaries
C. if treated surgically is usually followed with chemotherapy
D. has had a decreased incidence since introduction of the cervical screening programme in the UK
E. can present with true incontinence

29. Polycystic ovarian syndrome

A. is also known as Stein–Curtis syndrome
B. may be treated with clomiphene
C. may present with alopecia
D. is associated with raised LH and FSH levels
E. commonly presents with menorrhagia

30. Regarding partograms

A. the slowest acceptable rate of progress in a multiparous woman is 1 cm every 2 hours
B. if delay occurs in the second stage in a primigravida, oxytocin must not be used
C. if delay occurs at 7 cm in a multiparous woman inefficient uterine action is the commonest cause
D. they are graphic descriptions of labour
E. they are only useful if vaginal examinations are documented every 2 hours

Answers

1. A – T   Vaginal candidiasis can be transmitted to the fetus at
the time of vaginal delivery

       B – F   *Gardnerella vaginalis* is *discouraged* by an increase in
the number of döderleins bacilli in the vagina, as the
latter act to lower the pH of the vagina

       C – F   vaginal candidiasis is treated by local therapy, e.g.
clotrimazole pessaries or oral therapy, e.g. fluconazole

       D – F   metronidazole can be given throughout pregnancy but
as with all drugs is best avoided in the first trimester

       E – T   gonorrhoea can cause bartholinitis, cervicitis,
urethritis, pelvic and inflammatory disease

2. A – F   cervical polyps do not cause miscarriage

       B – T   cervical polyps can cause bleeding at any time either in
the nonpregnant or pregnant state. The majority,
however, are asymptomatic

       C – F   water discharge is usually due to infection or very
rarely tubal carcinoma; it would be a most unusual
presentation for a cervical polyp

       D – F   cervical polyps are covered by columnar epithelium

       E – T   cervical polyps can cause both intermenstrual and
postcoital bleeding

3. A – F   an enterocoele is a prolapse of the pouch of Douglas
which may contain bowel or omentum and does not
affect bladder function

       B – F   pelvic floor exercises may improve stress incontinence.
Bladder drill is more useful in the patient with
detrusor instability

       C – T   upper motor neurone lesions are associated with a
hyper-reflexic or so called 'neuropathic' bladder

       D – F   urodynamics should be performed in all women with
incontinence. Symptoms of stress incontinence may be
caused by detrusor contractions

       E – T   any mass in the pelvis can cause acute urinary
retention, including retained blood in the vagina
secondary to an imperforate hymen

4. A – **T**   if there is a large cystocoele and significant uterine prolapse there may be persistent residual urine in the bladder following voiding

      B – **F**   African women rarely suffer uterovaginal prolapse, the reason for this remaining uncertain

      C – **F**   a Hodge pessary is used for anteversion of a retroverted uterus. A ring or shelf pessary may be used for uterine prolapse

      D – **F**   an enlarged uterus is not a predisposing factor

      E – **F**   the factor contributing most to utero-vaginal prolapse is childbirth, so premenopausal women can have this problem, although the condition may deteriorate when the tissues become oestrogen deficient with ovarian failure

5. A – **F**   a 'double' (didelphic) uterus acts as a single uterus. It is the more subtle Müllerian duct abnormalities (e.g. arcuate uterus) that result in abnormal presentations

      B – **T**   multiple pregnancies have a higher incidence of transverse lie and all other malpresentations

      C – **F**   the commonest presentation of a second twin is cephalic, followed by a breech

      D – **T**   if the placenta is in the lower segment or overlying the cervix, i.e. placenta praevia, there will be an increased chance of a transverse lie

      E – **F**   in the presence of ruptured membranes and a preterm fetus a classical Caesarean section may be necessary but each case must be considered individually. At term the transverse fetus is usually delivered at Caesarean section by bringing the legs down and out of the wound first

6. A – **F**   substandard care was evident in nearly 50% of the reported cases of direct and indirect deaths

      B – **F**   the main causes of direct maternal deaths were thrombosis and thromboembolism, hypertensive disorders and haemorrhage

      C – **T**   guidelines have been issued with regard to the management of major obstetric haemorrhage. These include prompt and adequate fluid replacement and *senior* assistance

D – T deaths due to anaesthesia had decreased, in part related to the use of epidurals and spinals as opposed to general anaesthesia

E – T figures reported in this trienium were for the United Kingdom as a whole but comment was made regarding the lower rate in Ireland

7. A – F if estrogen replacement therapy is given in conjunction with 12 days of progestagen therapy, the incidence of carcinoma of the endometrium is decreased

B – T an endometrial biopsy will provide an histological diagnosis

C – F treatment is usually a total abdominal hysterectomy with bilateral salpingo-oophorectomy and may be followed by radiotherapy depending on the depth of endometrial involvement

D – F obese women have more conversion of androgen precursors to oestrone and so have a higher incidence

E – T endometrial hyperplasia without atypia carries a small risk (around 2%) of developing malignancy, but the presence of atypical cells increases the risk

8. A – T correct management of the third stage involves placing a hand suprapubically to prevent inversion of the uterus when the placenta is delivered. However, the aetiology in some women remains uncertain

B – T placenta accreta or percreta must be considered in the presence of uterine inversion

C – F removal of an attached placenta in this situation may cause uncontrollable bleeding

D – T if initial manual attempts at replacing the uterus have failed, then the hydrostatic method is used

E – F replacement should be attempted as soon as uterine inversion occurs by placing a fist beneath the inverted fundus and pushing cephalad. If this procedure is delayed then oedema of the tissues occurs making replacement even more difficult

9. A – **F**   unilateral enlargement can be due to a hydrocoele of the canal of *Nuck*

B – **T**   pox virus (*Molluscum contagiosum*), as with other viral infections (herpes, warts), can cause itchy vulva

C – **T**   testosterone cream (2%) may be of value in atrophic vulval lesions. Commonly aqueous cream or hydrocortisone ointments are tried initially

D – **F**   vulval carcinoma forms about 5% of all genital tract cancers

E – **T**   because of this rather embarrassing complaint, presentation is often delayed. Physicians should also not hesitate to inspect the vulva, prior to prescribing topical therapy

10. A – **T**   chronic ectopic pregnancies can present in this way

B – **F**   urinary pregnancy tests may be negative in ectopic pregnancy, therefore serum β-HCG should be measured. Where this service is not available, the case should be managed on clinical grounds

C – **T**   an incomplete miscarriage may present with a history of this nature. The diagnosis is often made by ultrasound; if the clinical findings are not conclusive

D – **F**   this phrase is only infrequently used now. It was thought to apply to a shortened luteal phase (less than 10 days) and low peak serum progesterone secondary to inadequate follicular development. Proof of its existence, however, is almost impossible

E – **T**   prolonged bleeding due to hormonal causes will usually respond to high-dose progestagens. Alternatively oestrogens can be tried

11. A – **F**   all normal term babies will lose up to 10% of their birthweight in the first few days of life; however, birthweight should be regained by 7–*10* days

B – **T**   babies with inborn errors of metabolism should not be breastfed as they require specifically artificially manipulated feeds

C – **F**   erythema toxicum (urticaria neonatorum) occurs in the first week of life and is of uncertain cause but harmless

D – **F**   physiological jaundice commences on days 2–4 of life and is due to increased unconjugated bilirubin levels. Onset of jaundice in the first 24 hours of life is abnormal and requires investigation

E – **T**   oxygen administration in preterm infants can cause retrolental fibroplasia and in severe cases can lead to blindness

12. A – **F**   there is no treatment for azoospermia unless it is due to a vasectomy, in which case re-anastomosis of the vas deferens may be successful

B – **F**   no WBCs are normally seen in a semen sample

C – **T**   a maximum of up to 50% of abnormal forms are acceptable in a semen sample

D – **F**   testicular failure produces high FSH and LH levels

E – **T**   micromanipulation allows easier entry of the spermatozoon into the zygote. Its usefulness has been proven in cases of poorly motile sperm

13. A – **F**   laparoscopies have a mortality of approximately 1 in 15,000, although this may vary with the increasing use of laparoscopic surgery

B – **F** CO_2 embolus is a complication which can occur in laparoscopy. This gas is used to insufflate the abdomen through a verres needle

C – **T** CO_2 left in the abdominal cavity can irritate the diaphragm postoperatively and cause shoulder-tip pain via the phrenic nerve

D – **T**   the bladder must be empty before insertion of the verres needle

E – **T**   peritoneal infection can result from laparoscopies by direct introduction of bacteria, by damaging internal organs or by injecting dye through the cervix into the upper genital tract

14. A – **T**   the large differences in various populations may have been exaggerated by selection bias. In the USA and England rates of incidence between 0.5–2 per 1000 pregnancies have been reported

B – **T**   the uterus may be larger, equivalent or smaller than expected for the expected gestation

C – T   vaginal bleeding is the most common presenting symptom. Theca lutein ovarian cysts are not infrequent and associated with hyperemesis and pre-eclampsia

D – F   regional centres (Charing Cross Hospital in London) operate a computerized follow-up system. Patients are contacted direct and urine or serum samples for β-HCG sent through the post

E – T   following any subsequent pregnancy HCG levels should be estimated to ensure that they have fallen to insignificant levels

15. A – F   as with all cases of collapse the priorities are Airway, Breathing and Circulation

B – T   as thromboplastin is released into the circulation, DIC rapidly develops and may be impossible to correct

C – F   the most likely cause is an atonic uterus; a cervical tear is rare. A systematic approach to the patient ensures that all possibilities are investigated

D – F   a uterine dehiscence should always be thought of in a woman with a previous Caesarean section

E – T   pregnant women have an increased incidence of thromboembolism regardless of the mode of delivery

16. A – F   women with Turner's syndrome have normal external female genitalia

B – F   in testicular feminization the phenotype is female but the gentotype contains a Y chromosome and testes are present

C – F   in cryptorchidism the testes have failed to descend and may be in the inguinal canal, but the external genitalia are male

D – T   the adrenogenital syndrome is the commonest cause of intersex and is caused by a female fetus being exposed to an excess of adrenal androgens

E – F   Kleinfelter's syndrome is a chromosomal disorder with 47XXY composition. The genitalia are male

17. A – **T** because of the increase in plasma volume (approximately 50% in primiparas and 60% in multigravidae) the actual values of electrolytes decrease

B – **F** the mucoid discharge from the cervix *increases* in pregnancy

C – **F** the respiratory tidal volume increases, as does the pulmonary blood flow

D – **T** cardiac output rises in the first trimester and continues to rise until it plateaus at around 34 weeks gestation

E – **F** in pregnancy a fasting blood glucose less than 5.8 mmol/L is normal and unchanged from the pre-pregnant state

18. A – **F** in severe pre-eclampsia the creatinine clearance rate is reduced

B – **T** the second wave of trophoblastic invasion to form the placental microcirculation is thought to be defective in women with severe PET

C – **T** there is an increased incidence of placental abruption, the placenta itself having reduced perfusion secondary to vasoconstriction

D – **F** the intravascular compartment is *decreased*

E – **T** all levels of electrolytes are increased because the fluid volume in the intravascular compartment is decreased. Rising serum urate levels are used to monitor the disease process

19. A – **F** once significant antibodies are present there is no point in giving anti-D

B – **T** amniocentesis can cause rhesus sensitization and therefore 250 IU of anti-D are given intramuscularly to rhesus-negative women (at 20 weeks or less of gestation)

C – **F** anti-D is not given routinely in early pregnancy to rhesus-negative women although it should always be given after a miscarriage or ectopic pregnancy

D – **F** the Kleihauer test may not be sensitive enough to pick up a very small transfer of fetal cells into the maternal circulation

E – F   the ABO incompatibility does not influence initiation of rhesus disease

20. A – F   engagement is defined as when the maximum diameter of the head (the biparietal diameter) has passed through the pelvic brim

      B – F   engagement is determined by the abdominal findings as the vaginal level of the presenting part is altered by moulding and therefore is an unreliable finding

      C – T   engagement is defined as when the maximum diameter of the head (the biparietal diameter) has passed through the pelvic brim

      D – T   in abdominal palpation, engagement is defined as 0/5, 1/5 or 2/5 of the head palpable above the pelvic brim

      E – F   it is the bony parts of the fetal head that are of importance, not the oedema and swelling of the soft tissues of the scalp (caput succedaneum)

21. A – T   in addition to the surge of follicle stimulating hormone there is a surge in luteinizing hormone, the detection of which is used in commercial urine ovulation detector kits

      B – T   as a result of ovulation, the endometrium changes from proliferative to secretory

      C – F   following ovulation the cervical mucus becomes less fluid and more viscous. It helps prevent the ascent of organisms and sperm to the upper genital tract

      D – T   the basal body temperature rises by approximately 0.3°C following ovulation and remains high throughout the secretory phase

      E – T   the second half of the menstrual cycle is usually constant and is 14 days from ovulation to menstruation. The proliferative phase of the endometrium cycle can vary

22. A – F   as oestrogen is metabolized through the liver oral therapy will cause a decrease in antithrombin III. Therefore a woman with past history of thromboembolic disease should be given parenteral

therapy, e.g. transdermal or implants
B – **T** premarin 0.625 mg has been shown to be bone sparing
C – **F** cystic hyperplasia can be treated medically by giving 12 days of progestagens each month. Repeated endometrial biopsy is warranted
D – **F** an endometrial thickness greater than 5 mm on ultrasound examination is significant
E – **F** oestrogen replacement therapy will *increase* HDL levels

23. A – **F** if a breech is to be delivered vaginally then oxytocin should not be used
B – **F** extraction should never normally be employed. The accoucheur merely guides the delivery of the fetus which is occuring by uterine contractions and maternal effort
C – **T** this is the widest dimension of the presenting part in a 'frank' or extended breech. It accounts for approximately two-thirds of vaginal breech deliveries
D – **T** in addition to the risks of prematurity, the fetus presenting by the breech has a higher rate of congenital abnormality and antepartum stillbirth than those with vertex presentation
E – **F** it is important to keep the fetal back anteriorly otherwise the chin may become caught on the symphysis pubis causing extension of the head and obstruct delivery

24. A – **F** the latest triennial report (1988–1990) and the maternal mortality rate for the past two reports has been 10 per 100 000 total births
B – **F** deaths related to hypertension are most commonly caused by intracerebral haemorrhage
C – **T** Mendelssohn's syndrome is aspiration of gastric contents and this most commonly occurs after emergency general anaesthesia rather than an elective general or epidural anaesthetic
D – **T** the incidence of death from pulmonary embolism (PE) after Caesarean section has fallen during the last twenty years but not the actual number of deaths. The

reason for this is that the incidence of PE's themselves has decreased, but there are more Caesarean sections performed

E – **F**   it is very difficult to prevent amniotic fluid embolism

25. A – **T**   hyperprolactinaemia can cause infertility and amenorrhoea. A serum prolactin estimation is an important baseline investigation, even in the woman without galactorrhoea

B – **F**   hyperprolactinaemia is treated with dopamine *agonist* drugs, most commonly bromocriptine

C – **T**   laboratory limits vary and some set the upper limit of normal unrealistically low. The level also increases with stress, eating, nipple stimulation, during sleep, intercourse and anaesthesia

D – **T**   hyperprolactinaemia can be physiological during pregnancy and breast feeding

E – **F**   a microadenoma or adenoma of the anterior pituitary gland is often found

26. A – **F**   placebo response rates are in the region of 90%, hence the utmost importance of placebo control in any therapeutic trial

B – **T**   success has been reported by eating frequent meals, reducing sugar and salt intake and cutting out caffeine sources

C – **T**   a symptom diary together with menstrual dates over the course of 2–3 months is important to exclude a symptom pattern not in agreement with PMS

D – **T**   the combined oral contraceptive and luteinizing hormone releasing hormone (LHRH) agonists have been successfully used in this role

E – **F**   controlled trials have shown this drug to be successful in improving the symptoms of fatigue, depression, headache, tension and irritability

27. A – **T**   palmar rash is a sign of secondary syphilis, together with the symptoms of fever, headache, bone and joint pains

B – F   the primary chancre of syphilis heals after 5–8 *weeks*

C – F   condylomata acuminata are warts caused by human papilloma virus, condylomata lata are the classical lesion of *secondary* syphilis

D – F   it is with *secondary* disease that the regional lymph nodes become active

E – F   secondary syphilis is highly infective

28.   A – T   carcinoma of the cervix can be asymptomatic, or be associated with intermenstrual, postcoital or postmenopausal bleeding

B – T   stage 1b can be treated with Wertheim's hysterectomy with removal or conservation of the ovaries, depending on the clinical setting and the age of the patient

C – F   adjuvant therapy in carcinoma of the cervix is radiotherapy

D – F   the introduction of the cervical screening programme in the UK unfortunately has not decreased the incidence of cervical carcinoma. The rate in younger women (less than 40) is increasing

E – T   if a fistula develops following local infiltration then true urinary incontinence can occur

29.   A – F   polycystic ovarian syndrome is also known as Stein–*Leventhal* syndrome; the clinical symptoms are hirsutism, menstrual problems and obesity

B – T   if the patient wants to conceive she may respond to oral clomiphene citrate therapy

C – F   if the patient's serum testosterone is raised *hirsutism* may be the presenting complaint

D – F   although the plasma LH level is usually increased the FSH level is low or normal. A follicular phase LH to FSH ratio should be 3 to 1 or more

E – F   women with polycystic ovarian syndrome present with oligoamenorrhoea rather than menorrhagia

30.   A – F   the slowest acceptable rate of progress in a primigravida woman is 1 cm every hour and in a multiparous woman 2 cm every hour

B – **F**   the commonest cause of delay in labour in a
primigravida woman is inefficient uterine action and
oxytocin can be safely used, even in the second stage,
once the patient has been assessed

C – **F**   in a multiparous woman delay at 7 cm often implies
obstructed labour

D – **T**   a partogram is a graphic description of labour. Its
visual nature conveys much information at a glance

E – **F**   vaginal examinations are normally performed hourly to
four hourly depending on the unit's policy. It is
important that each is documented accurately,
together with descent of the head, as palpated per
abdomen

Case Studies

Note: in the following case studies, the answers are coded **+** for a definitely correct response, **−** for a definitely incorrect response, and **?** for a dubious response.

Case Study One: Management of Pre-eclampsia

The patient is a 26-year-old primigravida who has attended antenatal clinic regularly. At 32 weeks gestation her blood pressure is recorded as 140/95 and her urine test shows proteinuria (+2).

Which of the following are the most important to note?

A. *Non-pregnant blood pressure*
B. *Booking blood pressure*
C. *Previous history of renal disease*
D. *Abnormal weight gain/loss*
E. *Family history of pre-eclampsia*

A. **+** This is an important base-line record. In this case the patient's non-pregnant blood pressure is entered as 120/80.

B. **+** This is an important base-line record, especially if recorded in the first 20 weeks of pregnancy. In this case the patient's booking blood pressure is entered as 110/70.

C. **?** A history of renal disease, unless associated with other diseases, will prove of significance only if the patient goes on to develop severe pre-eclampsia. In this case there is no history of renal disease.

D. **?** Abnormal weight gain could be an important factor to note. In this case the patient has gained 3 kg over the last two weeks.

E. **?** Over recent years there has been some discussion on the possibility of there being a familial trait in pre-eclampsia but as yet there is no hard evidence to support this theory. In this case the patient does not know the family history in this regard.

On the evidence to hand would you admit this patient?

A. Yes
B. No

A. **+** B. **−**

The patient should be admitted to hospital. She is showing signs of early onset of pre-eclampsia, exhibiting significant proteinuria, and requires 48-hour monitoring of her blood pressure and assessment of her condition.

When examining the patient which do you consider could prove most helpful in assessing her condition?

A. General look of the patient
B. Optic fundi
C. Oedema
D. Reflexes
E. Abdomen
F. Liver

A. **?** The general look of the patient could be helpful; patients with pre-eclampsia may have vasoconstriction and tend not to have the 'glow' (vasodilation) of the normally pregnant woman. In this case the patient looks generally unwell.

B. **+** It is important to examine the optic discs for signs of raised intracranial pressure. In this case there is no abnormality.

C. **?** Some oedema is normal in pregnancy, but generalized or gross oedema is significant. This patient has generalized oedema and she says her hands, feet and face become worse in the evening.

D. **+** Reflexes are a good indicator; hyper-reflexia and sustained clonus are associated with pre-eclampsia. This patient is found to be hyper-reflexic but there is no clonus.

E. **+** It is important to examine the abdomen to assess growth of the fetus and presentation. In this patient the fundus is measured as 28 cm and the fetus is in breech presentation. The liquor volume appears reduced.

F. **?** In severe disease the liver could be affected but in this patient no abnormality is found.

Having examined the patient which investigations would you now carry out?

A. *Full blood count*
B. *Serum calcium*
C. *Clotting studies*
D. *Urea and creatinine*
E. *Serum urate*
F. *24-hour urine collection*
G. *Blood pressure*
H. *Ultrasound scan*
I. *Liver function tests*

A. **+** Hb: 13.8 g/dl – PCV: 0.37 – platelets: 175×10^9/L
B. **−** Serum calcium has no predictive value in pre-eclampsia.
C. **+** Clotting studies: normal
D. **+** Urea and creatinine: normal
E. **+** Serum urate: 0.35 mmol/L
F. **+** The 24-hour collection was found to contain 0.9 g protein a day
G. **+** Blood pressure is measured every 4 hours over 48 hours. This patient's blood pressure was recorded between 140/95 and 150/100 over the 48 hours.
H. **+** Ultrasound shows reduced liquor volume; abdominal circumference on the 5th percentile. Head circumference and femur length are normal.
I. **+** Liver function tests are normal.

How would you classify this patient's pre-eclampsia?

A. Mild
B. Moderate
C. Severe

A. — B. + C. ?

This patient's pre-eclampsia condition can be classified as moderate. Severe PET would require a higher blood pressure level, more proteinuria or other significant signs.

Would you discharge this patient at the end of her 48-hour assessment?

A. Yes
B. No

A. — B. +

This patient is showing signs of moderately severe pre-eclampsia and must be kept in hospital.

How often would you now repeat the haematological investigations?

A. Daily
B. Every 3 days
C. Weekly

A. — B. + C. —

Every three days is the optimum period.

Three days following the first investigations the results now show:
Blood pressure: stable
Proteinuria: 1.3 g in 24 hours
Hb: 13.8 g/dl
Platelets: 160×10^9/L
Clotting studies: normal
Serum urate: 0.39 mmol/L

The patient's urine is tested by dipstick daily and the proteinuria rises from +2 on the third day to +4 on the sixth day when the other investigations show:
Blood pressure: 140/110
Hb: 13.6 g/dl
Packed cell volume: 0.42
Platelets: 80×10^9/L
Serum urate: 0.42 mmol/L
Clotting studies: normal
Proteinuria: 5 g in 24 hours

On examination the patient looks worse, she has facial oedema and complains of a headache. She still has hyper-reflexia which is associated with 3 beats of clonus at the ankles.

Which would you prescribe for this patient? (select in order of priority)

A. Sedatives
B. Antihypertensives
C. Anticonvulsants
D. Diuretics
E. None

A. − Sedatives are contra-indicated as they will not improve the maternal disease process. Additionally, these drugs readily cross the placenta and could adversely affect the fetus which is already at risk.

B. + The immediate aim of management at this stage is to gain control of the blood pressure and so protect the cerebral vessels. Hydralazine is a non-specific vasodilator also useful for acute reduction of blood pressure and may be given intravenously as a bolus titrated against the blood pressure. The β-blocker labetalol has also been shown to be safe. Caution must be exercised in the asthmatic patient. Nifedipine is a calcium channel blocker and vasodilator and is widely used in this situation: it is taken sublingually (10 mg) and may worsen her headache.

C. **+** As a general rule the role of anticonvulsants is difficult to define in pre-eclampsia. If the patient feels quite well she is unlikely to have a fit and hyper-reflexia can be used as a guide, but it is not reliable; however, if clonus is present eclampsia is imminent. In this case the patient feels unwell and clonus is also present so an anticonvulsant such as intravenous phenytoin or magnesium sulphate should be given.

D. **–** Diuretics are contra-indicated.

E. **?**

The patient responds well to treatment and her blood pressure falls to 140/90. Which do you consider the better option for this patient and her baby?

A. *Monitor closely and try to delay delivery until the fetus is bigger*
B. *Deliver immediately*

A. **–** B. **+**

It would be dangerous to postpone delivery which is in effect, the definitive treatment of pre-eclampsia.

As the fetus is in breech position it is decided to opt for Caesarean section. Which anaesthetic technique would you choose?

A. *Epidural*
B. *General anaesthesia*

A. – B. +

The patient should have a general anaesthetic carefully administered by a senior skilled anaesthetist. Epidural anaesthesia is contra-indicated if the platelet count has fallen below 100, and this patient's count is 80. However, this is a controversial subject and some would perform a regional block (spinal) with normal clotting despite the patient's platelet count, the smaller needle making the risk of haematoma less. General anaesthesia increases systemic blood pressure and pulmonary capillary wedge pressure at induction – an unwanted effect in this situation.

What problems are most likely to occur when delivering this patient at 32 weeks?

A. *Difficult delivery*
B. *Haemorrhage*
C. *Fetal respiratory difficulties*

A. **?** Delivery may present problems at 32 weeks. The lower segment may be poorly formed and an inadequate uterine incision may cause difficulty because of entrapment of the after coming head.

B. **?** As this patient has a low platelet count there could be difficulties with haemostasis.

C. **+** Delivering the child at 32 weeks could result in respiratory difficulties.
   How could the problem be minimized?

   a. *Alert neonatal intensive care in advance*
   b. *Administer steroids to mother, ideally 24–48 hours prior to the delivery*
   c. *Administer endotracheal surfactant to the mother*

a. **+** b. **+** c. **–**

Although alerting the special care baby unit will help the infant, the administration of steroids to the mother when it becomes clear that an early delivery will be necessary will promote lung maturity. Artificial surfactant has been shown to be effective in reducing the incidence of infant respiratory distress. It is administered to the fetus once delivered, not to the mother.

The patient is delivered of a 1.1 kg infant; for how long following delivery would you maintain the patient on her drug regime of nifedipine and phenytoin?

A. *Stop medication immediately*
B. *Continue for 24 hours*
C. *Continue for 48 hours*
D. *Stop once the patient has passed 60 ml of urine in an hour*

A. − B. ? C. + D. −

The patient should be maintained on phenytoin for 48 hours following delivery as she is still at risk from eclampsia during this period. She is also likely to remain hypertensive and antihypertensive medication should be titrated against her blood pressure until it falls to normal levels. Fluid management with hourly urine output and central venous pressure (CVP) line is also important at this time.

The patient's urine output is measured at 40 ml/h increasing to 70 ml/h over 12 hours. Her blood pressure returns to normal levels within 48 hours and she, and her baby, make a good recovery.

Case Study Two: Breech Presentation

The patient is a fit and well primigravida aged 26. After missing antenatal clinic for a month, she next attends at 37 weeks when she is found to have a fundal height of 36 cm and breech presentation. On examination the head is lying towards the midline.

Would you perform external cephalic version (ECV)?

A. Yes
B. No

A. ? B. −

This is a controversial area and there is no role for using excessive force or performing it under general anaesthetic. In the past the fetus used to be turned to a cephalic presentation at 32–36 weeks. Randomized trials have shown that ECV at term significantly reduces the incidence of breech presentation at birth.

As ECV carries a small risk of placental abruption and cord accident many obstetricians do not attempt it.

What are the causes of breech presentation?

A. Uterine anomalies
B. Placental abruption
C. Fetal abnormality
D. Pre-eclampsia
E. Placenta praevia
F. Grand multiparity

A. **+** Uterine anomalies such as fibroids or bicornate uterus can cause breech presentation.

B. **−** Although the aetiology of placental abruption is unknown there is no particular association with breech presentation.

C. + Fetal abnormalities such as hydrocephalus or neural tube defect are associated with breech presentation.

D. − There is no association between pre-eclampsia and breech presentation.

E. + Placenta praevia is often found with breech presentation.

F. + Breech presentation is common in grand multiparity when the uterus can become lax

What investigations could prove most helpful in managing this patient?

A. *Ultrasound scan*
B. *Erect lateral pelvimetry*
C. *X-ray of fetus*

A. + Ultrasound is very useful; it will give information on fetal abnormality, placental position, assess liquor volume, estimate fetal weight and reveal the type of breech presentation: flexed leg (complete) or extended leg (frank).

In this case the scan shows a cornual placenta and an extended leg breech presentation. The liquor is normal and there is no fetal abnormality. The estimated fetal weight is 2.7 kg.

B. + X-ray pelvimetry is important as it will check that the mother's pelvis is of adequate size. The antero-posterior (AP) diameter of the pelvic inlet from behind the posterior edge at the top of the pubic symphysis to the sacral promentary should be greater than 11.5 cm. In this case the diameter is 12.5 cm.

C. ? An X-ray of the fetus is largely redundant as any information revealed by this method may be acquired by other, more valuable investigations and mother and child should not be exposed to unnecessary radiation.

From the evidence to hand do you consider this patient is suitable for vaginal delivery?

A. Yes
B. No

A. **+** B. **–**

As this patient's pelvic diameter is more than 11.5 cm, it is an extended leg breech, the fetus has no abnormality and is estimated to be of a favourable weight, vaginal delivery should be tried. It is important to counsel the parents and obtain their consent to the decision.

It is decided to opt for vaginal delivery; would you induce labour?

A. Yes
B. No

A. **–** B. **+**

It is better to wait for a spontaneous onset of labour as this has the best prognosis in terms of achieving a successful vaginal delivery.

During the discussions on her management the patient is anxious to know what pain relief she might have. How would you advise her?

A. Epidural
B. Pethidine
C. Inhaled 'gas and air'
D. Acupuncture

A. **+** Epidural anaesthesia would probably be the best choice for this patient as forceps are likely to be needed to control delivery of the aftercoming head and there is also an increased chance of a Caesarean section being required.

71

B. **?** If the patient is unwilling to undergo epidural anaesthesia then pethidine could be the next best choice as this narcotic is a powerful analgesic. However, it is not always effective, having a 40% failure rate, and has a high incidence of side-effects such as dizziness, nausea and vomiting, drowsiness, dissociated state of consciousness and hypotension.

C. − The inhalational agent, Entonox, consists of 50% nitrous oxide, 50% oxygen and has no harmful side-effects on either mother or child. It is self-administered and the mother has the advantage of control; however, it takes 20–30 seconds of inhalation to reach sufficient analgesia.

D. − Acupuncture, along with other physical methods such as massage or transcutaneous electrical nerve stimulation (TENS), is non-invasive and has no harmful effects on the fetus but is really only effective in the early stage of labour.

It is very important for the various options in pain relief to be fully discussed with the patient so that she can make her choice according to her own individual attitude. In this case she elects to have epidural anaesthesia.

The patient is admitted to the labour ward two weeks later at 39 weeks; she has had contractions for 3 hours, coming at the rate of 4 contractions in 10 minutes.

On vaginal examination the cervix is found to be 3 cm dilated with a buttock at 1 cm above the ischial spines. The membranes are ruptured.

The patient appears to be making normal progress. What else should be done at this stage?

A. *Apply fetal scalp electrode*
B. *Insert IV line*
C. *Administer an epidural*
D. *Augment with oxytocin infusion*

A. **?** If a poor external trace is limiting fetal monitoring a fetal scalp electrode should be applied to the buttock. Care should be taken to avoid the genitalia.

B. **+** An IV line should be inserted.

C. **+** The anaesthetist should administer the epidural at this stage.

D. **−** In the presence of good progress (greater than 1 cm per hour of cervical dilation) and with a breech presentation there is no role for oxytocin.

The patient progresses to full dilatation over the next 4 hours and spontaneous descent of the breech is allowed. One hour later the buttocks distend the perineum.

What factors are important in the delivery itself?

A. *Effectively topped up epidural*
B. *Anaesthetist present*
C. *Paediatrician present*
D. *Experienced obstetrician*
E. *Kielland's forceps*
F. *Intravenous oxytocin infusion*
G. *Applying traction to the groin*

A. **+** Fully effective epidural block is of great assistance for any instrumentation or manipulation that is required for delivery of the head.

B. **+** The presence of an anaesthetist is required in case it is necessary to resort to a Caesarean section.

C. **+** Paediatric support may be needed for resuscitation of the infant.

D. **+** A breech presentation is a high-risk delivery requiring senior obstetric support.

E. — Kielland's forceps have no role in this situation, but Neville Barnes (or other lift-out forceps) may be used for delivery of the after-coming head.

F. — The basic principle of a breech delivery is for the breech to be delivered spontaneously. There is no place for oxytocin with failure of descent.

G. — Groin traction would not be appropriate and merely risks extending the fetal arms and head.

The baby was delivered safely and without incident. Both mother and child followed a normal course and were discharged from hospital two days later.

Case Study Three: Abnormal Bleeding

A 34-year-old mother of two children attends gynaecological outpatient clinic complaining of protracted erratic vaginal bleeding.

Which of these aspects of the patient's history do you consider could be important?

A. *Duration of symptoms*
B. *Presence of intermenstrual bleeding*
C. *Post-coital bleeding and date of last smear*
D. *Contraceptive method*
E. *Previous and current treatment*
F. *Age of menarche*
G. *Presence or absence of dysmenorrhoea*

A. **?** Duration of symptoms is not necessarily a good guide for diagnosing the cause of disturbances in menstrual pattern. GPs vary widely in their criteria for referral, with some referring after just one abnormal period, whilst others will wait for years before sending the patient to hospital.

B. **+** Intermenstrual bleeding should always be taken seriously. Its presence is often an indication for endometrial sampling and hysteroscopy.

C. **+** Post-coital bleeding may suggest a local cause for the irregular blood loss. The date and result of the last smear is very important.

D. **+** It is important to know if the patient is using contraception as it is possible the bleeding could be pregnancy related, i.e. retained products of conception.
The 'mini-pill' is a known cause of erratic vaginal bleeding in approximately one-third of the women who take it; others experience amenorrhoea and some regular monthly bleeds. Inert intrauterine contraceptive devices are associated with an increase in the volume of menstrual blood loss.

E. **+** The patient's past and current treatment can be established from both the GP's referral letter and questioning of the patient. In this instance the patient has not received any previous treatment.

F. **−** The patient's age of menarche is unlikely to bear any relevance to her current symptoms. We can confidently assume she has adequate reproductive function, as evidenced by her two children.

G. **?** Presence or absence of dysmenorrhoea could be of significance, but pain is not a predominant symptom in this patient.

The patient is experiencing menstrual bleeding with a cycle interval of 18–30 days; the duration of the menses varies between 8 and 11 days. There is no intermenstrual or post-coital loss. In this case the patient does have an intrauterine contraceptive device.

When examining the patient which features are most important to note?

A. *Presence of swollen ankles*
B. *Stigmata of anaemia*
C. *Signs of hypothyroidism*
D. *Presence of abdominal mass*
E. *Inspection of vagina, vulva and cervix*
F. *Bimanual palpation of the pelvic organs*

A. **−** Swollen ankles are unlikely to be of any direct relevance to this case.

B. **?** Although haemoglobin levels generally tend to fall with increasing menstrual bleeding, patients often compensate satisfactorily by eating an adequate diet and may have a haemoglobin within the normal range.

C. **+** It is uncommon to find hypothyroidism in women who first present with menstrual irregularity. However, this possibility should always be borne in mind. In this case, both the patient's history and clinical examination indicate that she is euthyroid.

D. **+** Before performing a vaginal examination an adequate abdominal examination is mandatory; it is surprisingly easy to overlook a large abdominal mass if this rule is broken. In this case no abnormal findings are found.

E. **+** Careful inspection of the vagina, vulva and cervix is important to exclude any local cause for erratic bleeding. On examination the entire area appears healthy. IUD strings are seen coming from the cervical os.

F. **+** Bimanual palpation is important in assessing the size, tenderness and mobility of the pelvic organs. In this instance the IUD strings were readily felt and the uterus found to be of normal size, anteverted, mobile, non-tender and with no associated adnexal masses.

The patient is counselled with regard to the various options available to her. It is suggested that the IUD be removed. She agrees and is happy to try an alternative method of contraception.

When removing the IUD which of these are most important to bear in mind?

A. Stage in menstrual cycle
B. Recent sexual intercourse
C. Husband's wishes
D. Type of IUD

A. **+** The fertile period in a woman with a regular 28-day cycle is 2–3 days around day 14, but in this particular instance the bleeding irregularity adds to the difficulties in establishing when ovulation may have occurred.

B. **+** It is very important to know if recent sexual intercourse has taken place; sperms have been known to survive for 5–7 days in the female reproductive tract. Possible implantation of a pregnancy following removal of the device should therefore be borne in mind.

C. **?** Contraception is usually a joint decision between both partners, but the variety of methods available mean that almost always a suitable alternative can be found.

D. **−** The type of IUD is irrelevant.

The patient is currently menstruating and has not had intercourse for the previous 14 days. A Nova-T is removed with ease using a Spencer−Wells forceps to pull the strings.

The patient is advised to keep a record of menstrual bleeding and to have her diaphragm refitted. No follow-up appointment is made but she is offered the option of returning to the clinic if not satisfied with the results of the intervention.

Subsequently the patient is seen in the hospital some two years later, delighted to be pregnant with her planned third baby. She comments that removal of the IUD had resulted in the restoration of an acceptable flow and regular menstrual bleeding, lasting only 3−5 days.

Case Study Four: Menorrhagia

A 45-year-old women attends the gynaecology clinic with a history of excessively heavy menstrual periods for the previous year. She has no menopausal symptoms.

When taking the history which of these factors could prove most valuable in influencing this patient's management?

A. *Disruption to life*
B. *Volume of blood loss*
C. *Episodes of flooding*
D. *Passage of clots*
E. *Number of sanitary items used*

A. **+** The patient is manageress of a local Building Society and because of uncontrollable menstrual flow she needs to take one or two days off work every month.

B. **+** Assessing the volume of menstrual bleeding in patients with menorrhagia is notoriously inaccurate. Approximately 50% of women who complain of excessively heavy periods will in fact have a blood loss of less than 80 ml per period, which is within the normal range. Objective menorrhagia is defined as a menstrual blood loss per period in excess of 80 ml. In practice, however, blood loss is rarely measured and clinicians rely on patients' subjective impressions.

C. **+** She has experienced several episodes of flooding while at work and the necessity to change sanitary protection at frequent intervals is making it impossible to work and therefore maintain her senior position at the branch.

D. **?** What is considered a clot is subjective, ranging from a tiny coagulum a few millimetres in diameter to the passage of clots the size of a fist.

E. **?** The amount of sanitary wear used is not an accurate indication of the volume of menstrual bleeding; it will vary according to fastidiousness, financial restrictions and the absorbency of these items.

The patient is experiencing 5 days of heavy flow, worst on days 2 and 3, at intervals of approximately 28 days. In addition, she has intermenstrual spotting at any time within the cycle.
Findings on examination are unremarkable, other than to note the scars from the laparoscopic clip sterilization of some 8 years ago.

Which investigations do you consider most appropriate?

A. *Urea and electrolytes*
B. *Full blood count*
C. *Hysteroscopy*
D. *Cervical smear*
E. *Endometrial sampling*

A. − Urea and electrolytes are of little relevance unless the patient has other evidence of systemic illness; the results are unlikely to influence the patient's management.

B. + Full blood count would be useful in checking whether the heavy menstrual flow has resulted in an anaemia. An iron deficiency picture may be present indicating the need for iron supplementation.

C. + Hysteroscopy is an important investigation in view of the intermenstrual bleeding. This procedure can be conducted in an outpatient setting without the need for general anaesthesia.

D. ? It is always important to establish how recently a cervical smear was obtained, in addition to inspecting the cervix.

E. + Endometrial sampling is indicated in this patient who is over 40 and experiencing intermenstrual bleeding and therefore has an increased risk of endometrial pathology.
    Dilatation and curettage is now usually performed in combination with hysteroscopy. Suspicious areas can then be specifically biopsied and any endometrial polyps removed.

There are no facilities available for outpatient hysteroscopy and the patient is therefore admitted for a D&C and hysteroscopy under general anaesthetic as a day case the following month.

On reviewing the procedure notes in outpatient clinic 6 weeks later to what should special attention be paid?

A. Clinical findings at examination under anaesthetic
B. Endometrial histology
C. Whether she is currently menstruating

A. **?** No unusual features were noted, in agreement with those established at her initial consultation.

B. **+** Chasing up the endometrial histology is important in excluding atypical hyperplasia or endometrial carcinoma.
　　　Endometrial sampling which has been performed in the latter part of the menstrual cycle could be expected to show secretory changes in a woman who is ovulating.

C. **−** Whether or not the patient is menstruating is not of importance.

The patient is found to have no cervical or intra-uterine polyps or other abnormality. The endometrial history showed normal secretory-phase endometrium, consistent with day 20 of the menstrual cycle.

What management option(s) would best benefit this patient?

A. Reassurance
B. Medical treatment
C. Surgery

A. **+** The patient can be reassured that there is no underlying sinister cause of her symptoms. She can be advised that she will, at some time, go through a spontaneous menopause when her problems will be resolved. However, she is unlikely to find this an acceptable solution, particularly in view of the detrimental effects menstruation is having on her career.

B. **+** Medical treatment has a number of advantages. Appropriate drug therapy can be expected to reduce menstrual flow by approximately 50%, although there is a variable response rate. In addition, it involves no risks from either general anaesthesia or surgery and it does not require any time spent in hospital or in recuperation. Ideally medical therapy should always be tried before resorting to surgery.

C. **?**

After counselling the patient elects to opt for trial of medical therapy.

Which of these drug therapies would you advise?

A. *Mefenamic acid*
B. *Paracetamol*
C. *Tranexamic acid*
D. *Progestagens*
E. *Danazol*
F. *Combined oral contraceptive*

A. **+** Mefenamic acid reduces menstrual flow by an average of 30% and is also effective in the relief of dysmenorrhoea.

B. **−** Paracetamol has no effect on the volume of menstrual bleeding.

C. **+** Tranexamic acid has the advantage of being taken only during the menstrual period and reduces the menstrual blood volume by approximately 50%.

D. **?** Progestagens taken as a short course during the luteal phase of the cycle are unlikely to be of great benefit in the ovulatory woman. However more extended courses (for example 20 days of the cycle) may be more beneficial and may have the additional advantage of preventing intermenstrual bleeding.

E. ? Danazol, taken at a dosage of 200 mg daily, is an effective medical method of reducing menstrual blood loss. This patient was unwilling to try it as her daughter had suffered side-effects when danazol had been prescribed at higher doses for endometriosis.

F. ? Combined oral contraceptives are an effective method for controlling the cycle and reducing menstrual blood flow. However this therapy is thought to be inappropriate in this case in view of the patient's age and her habit of smoking 5–10 cigarettes a day.

The patient is prescribed tranexamic acid 1 g qds with the menses for three months but she is unable to tolerate the tablets because of nausea.

She is then prescribed a course of progestagens for days 5–24 of her menstrual cycle and given an appointment for review in three months.

When the patient returns to clinic she has stopped taking her medicine as she could not tolerate the feeling of being 'bloated and depressed'.

She states a desire for surgery as an end to her menses.

Which surgical procedure would you advise?

A. Repeated D & C
B. Endometrial distruction
C. Vaginal hysterectomy
D. Total abdominal hysterectomy with bilateral salpingo-oopherectomy

A. − This procedure offers no long-term effect on the volume of bleeding although it was previously considered a 'cure'.

B. + A variety of minimally invasive techniques have been developed to remove the endometrium, including resection, laser ablation, thermal damage and radio frequency. These procedures have the advantages of a short hospital stay and shorter recuperation time than conventional surgery; however they cannot guarantee amenorrhoea.

C. **+** Vaginal hysterectomy has the advantages of guaranteeing amenorrhoea and removing both the cervix and endometrium, which are possible sites for carcinoma. In addition, the procedure is associated with less postoperative pain and less morbidity than abdominal surgery. Laparoscopic assisted vaginal hysterectomy has been suggested as a means of converting a procedure that formerly would only have been done at laparotomy per abdomen to a vaginal route.

D. **?** Abdominal hysterectomy is a major operation with significant morbidity and mortality. It does however guarantee amenorrhoea. It is important to discuss the issue of oopherectomy with the patient: the removal of the ovaries will prevent subsequent development of ovarian carcinoma. However, HRT will be necessary and should be continued until at least the age of natural menopause, both to protect the cardiovascular system and bones and prevent the unpleasant sequelae of a surgically induced menopause.

After consultation and counselling she opts for an endometrial resection.